'I su

trea

type

rept

grea

Yeh

'Zita

deve

preg

who

anyt

reco

Kate

'Kno

reas

Stell

'Preg

worr

ackn

need

treats

impo

nothi

even the most trivial fears. Over the years, Zita has become a true friend and her generosity and concern know no bounds.'

Ulrika Jonsson

'What Zita West doesn't know about being pregnant isn't worth knowing.'

Lucy Cavendish, *Evening Standard*

Client Quotes

'I feel like I have been transformed by the Zita West approach. It is such a relief at last to have a realistic plan of action and a clear focus on what I need to do to get pregnant.'

'It was so refreshing that the focus wasn't just on me, but on my partner as well. They really investigated the causes of our problems. Men aren't catered for in clinics as the focus is on one healthy sperm for ICSI. After doing the male health programme, my partner changed aspects of his lifestyle and diet. This led to a huge improvement which has resulted in my longed-for pregnancy!'

'I've been down so many routes in my quest to conceive and it's so refreshing to find somewhere that truly integrates a Western approach that works alongside complementary health. Zita's programme has been the perfect support for me and allayed my anxieties about pregnancy.'

'Zita's fertility awareness sessions have made me realize I was missing the window of opportunity to conceive as, having been on the pill for years, I never really understood my cycle. Her grounded commonsense approach helped me without making me feel embarrassed or inadequate. I conceived three months after visiting her clinic!'

'Zita's clinic and staff were a real haven of tranquillity to me in what was a very stressful IVF cycle. The support that I received really helped me to get through the difficult weeks.'

'Our baby boy was born last month. We couldn't be happier and it's thanks to all the help and guidance I got from Zita and her team. The words "Thank you" just don't seem enough.'

ZITA WEST'S GUIDE
TO GETTING
PREGNANT

Zita West

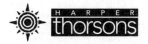
HARPER
thorsons

HarperThorsons
An Imprint of HarperCollins*Publishers*
77-85 Fulham Palace Road,
Hammersmith, London W6 8JB

The website address is:
www.thorsonselement.com

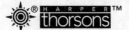

and *HarperThorsons* are trademarks of
HarperCollins*Publishers* Ltd

First published by HarperThorsons 2005

6

© Zita West 2005

A catalogue record of this book
is available from the British Library

ISBN-13 978-0-00-717371-6
ISBN-10 0-00-717371-7

Printed and bound in Great Britain by
Clays Ltd, St Ives plc

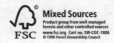

contents

dedication

I would like to dedicate this book to my mother for her help, guidance and support over the years in all I have achieved.

acknowledgements

I would especially like to thank:

Harriet Griffey for her help and enthusiasm with writing this book.

My husband for his endless patience.

The team in my clinic: Jane Knight, Melanie Brown, Maureen Kylie, Sheryl Homa, Jane Cassidy, Lindsey Taylor, Josephine Ceraq, Holly Dunbar, Cheween Lawes, Victoria Francis, Claire Norris, Liz Dick, Catherine Brown, Sally Anne Caplin, Anita O'Neill, Brian Astley, Jo Hill and Linda Rose.

For their helpful contributions: Claire Mellon, Karl Olah, Simon Rattenbury and Gerad Kite, Vicki McIvor, Wanda Whiteley, Simon Gerratt and all at Thorsons.

Barbara Vesey for her input and enthusiasm.

introduction

Information Overload!

Having a child is the most creative thing you can imagine but, for so many, the balance between what we are told to do as responsible parents and what we need to do to maintain an effective and enjoyable life in work and leisure seems to have gone. There are self-help books, theories, courses, experts, gurus galore, all with something to say, demanding attention. The driving aim of my work is to help couples to make sense of the maze – to gain a better understanding of where they are and how to move forward, practically – and it gives me the greatest pleasure.

Let's be realistic about modern life: Lots of men and women work long, stressful hours, particularly at the time of life when they are thinking of having children. They are bombarded with stimulation, information, expectations: it all leads to overload. So many couples have lost focus, running down many routes: Trying to conceive, undertaking all sorts of treatments, but often not looking at their everyday environment and things that they can do for *themselves*. Let's keep it simple.

The focus of many clinics and books like this is often wholly on the woman and her situation. But, as I'll point out, problems conceiving can equally be with the male partner. So in this book you will find me frequently talking about the health of both partners in a couple, and there is a lot of information about male fertility.

If you are going to take control of your own fertility, you need to understand it properly. This book offers you practical knowledge and information about how your fertility works, how to monitor it and how to help improve it. Many of my clients are extremely intelligent, high-achieving, successful people, but they are ignorant of the biological basics. It's something they are often acutely embarrassed about, but it's not entirely surprising – it's easy to get lost in all the medical jargon. However, hidden in that jargon is important information. Don't be tempted to just give up on it and flee to complementary treatments as an escape. The medicine we've got used to in Western countries is highly technical, and has perhaps become impersonal in its approach, but it can be used to extremely good effect. Good complementary approaches, particularly those that deal with the whole person – body, mind and spirit – can be very valuable, too, but it is important to choose the right ones, the right practitioners and, crucially, to combine them with a proper medical approach.

This book brings both approaches together, getting the best from each. It reflects the special aspect of the work I do every day in my own clinic – a truly integrated use of Western and complementary practice. Western medicine is evidence based and founded on proven measurable results. As far as possible, the treatments I advocate are equally evidence based, even in the area of complementary care.

More than that, I am interested in *why* couples want to have children; what else in their lives is making that possible or difficult; why perhaps they haven't thought about it before.

It is a fact that women are leaving it later to have children. There are many reasons for this trend, but there is no getting away from the fact that the chances of conception diminish with age. Being realistic, I firmly believe that women in their thirties should be fast tracked for investigation. They do not have indefinite time left to keep trying, and there may be fertility problems to be addressed.

Perhaps one of the reasons couples delay pregnancy is an increasing need and expectancy for perfection. They think, 'We'll just wait until next year for a better income/home/lifestyle' and so on. But of course the perfect moment never comes, even though there's an industry of self-help programmes guiding you towards that perfect balance. And then, as with 'perfect' diets, when you stray from the path there's often guilt and remorse to cope with and you have to start all over again. This book is not about being perfect, but about being practical.

Zita West

the way I work

Planning to get pregnant often follows other life plans – getting a longed-for job, finding a life partner, buying a first home – then comes having a baby. For some there comes a period in their lives where all the pieces of the jigsaw are in place, and the timing is right for having a baby. For others, there is an emphasis on getting everything 'just perfect' before ever considering having a baby.

Working with couples who are trying for a baby is multifaceted. Couples trying for a baby have many issues that are unique to them. I try and work with a couple to see their individual and unique whole picture.

Having said this, I believe there is no point in our lives when the timing is just right, and I wish I could encourage more couples not to set themselves unrealistic goals. Now I am a mother with a teenage daughter, it's only natural that I want her to get a good university degree, find a rewarding job and a steady relationship. I was 27 when I found myself pregnant with her, and was devastated at first. I did six pregnancy tests to check, because I had not 'planned' on having children until my thirties. Although I had been married for a while, my husband and I had no money and were working abroad, and I thought the timing was terrible. Now, I wouldn't have done it any other way!

Having been doing this work for the last 15 years, I found in the first few years that it was very much the woman in a partnership who would come along for the initial consultation; I would never see the partner. Nowadays I am delighted to say that I see couples together all the time – which is only as it should be, as the problem, statistically, usually has to do with women 50 per cent of the time and with men the other 50 per cent of the time.

The majority of couples don't have a problem conceiving, but if you have bought this book, maybe getting pregnant isn't happening for you as quickly as you would like and you are looking for some information and answers. No matter what route you take, I believe that *you can take control of your own fertility* – not hand it over to a doctor or fertility clinic. This is how I work with the women and men who come to see me. I don't give them a pre-set, 'one size fits all' formula. Each couple is unique, and while their emotional and physical well-being is my main concern, I don't *tell* them what to do. Together we work out what will work best for them. It is my hope that this book will help you do the same. I am really delighted that more and more clinics are starting to take on my work, particularly as of course not everyone can come to our clinic. My aim in this book is to help you to plan the best course of action for you, and to indicate the kind of treatments you should try to find in your own locality.

Keeping It Simple

Day after day I sit with couples who have experienced difficulties at every stage of the fertility process, from the pre-conceptual check-up to those who have battled with miscarriage or assisted conception. Each of these couples has the same goal: they want to have a baby. Some are more desperate than others, and with desperation comes a kind of vulnerability. Many couples are running down endless routes, trying every available therapy without any real focus.

Many come to me just as they are about to embark on their goal. They are still optimistic – and usually with good reason – and want reassurance about their approach to conception and what steps to take in adjusting their lifestyle, diet or activities. They prove how starting off on the right foot can make all the difference; I have seen the results, and have a clinic full of photos of smiling mothers and babies to prove it.

Others who come to see me have already pursued all sorts of ways to get pregnant, and know they are having problems. Sometimes just the process of being listened to and being asked the appropriate questions elicits that nugget of information that may be key to the outcome (which is why the questionnaire I use is so detailed).

For example, I see many, many couples who are just not having sex often enough. It's as simple as that, but just saying 'have more sex' wouldn't be helpful. Helping a couple take a really good look at their lifestyle can be a real turning-point in their whole approach to having a baby, demonstrating the need for a radical change in their priorities and for unqualified commitment. The baby is not just another 'must do' item to fit into their life-plan.

There are so many myths around nutrition, intimacy and sex (see Male and Female Fertility chapters). Many GPs and clinics don't ask enough about couples' sex lives; the usual question is 'Are you having regular sex?' But what is regular sex? Once every Sunday morning may be regular sex to you, but it doesn't help if you are ovulating on a Wednesday. Also, couples who are on different schedules, do shift work, travel a lot – these are all huge factors when you are trying to conceive. There can also be psychosexual problems, and naturally many couples are embarrassed to discuss such matters, particularly if their GP or clinician is not asking the right questions, of if he is not making them feel comfortable or even worthy of his complete attention.

It Takes Two

Basic knowledge about anatomy and physiology is one area that inevitably needs to be explored. Not the nuts and bolts of what goes where, but the details of a woman's fertility cycle, and what the implications are for ovulation and possible conception. This is why fertility awareness is so integral to the way I work. Spending a king's ransom on ovulation-predictor tests won't help if you think your cycle is 28 days when what is normal for you is a 35-day cycle. Many women have been on the Pill for a long time and have no idea what their normal cycle is; nevertheless they often feel embarrassed by discussions around basic biology, as they feel they ought to know all about it.

In my experience of looking after couples who are trying to get pregnant, I am convinced that the neglect of the man's role in conception has also confounded many of their attempts to have a baby. The man is very often badly neglected when it comes to assessing a couple's fertility. A quick, cursory look at the quality and quantity of his sperm is about all that's done in most fertility clinics, with all the emphasis focused – often wrongly – on the woman. There may also be a notion that the whole of a man's ego and masculinity is bound up in his sperm, making any possible criticism – or even discussion – of his effectiveness in this area an attack on his masculinity. Neglecting a man's role in the scheme of things is not helpful. The way I work places as much importance on the man's role in conception as the woman's, which is why the questionnaire I supply for men is just as detailed as the one for women.

A Holistic Approach

Many couples find my approach to be very different from a consultation with their GP or a fertility clinic. The physical checks they give to patients' reproductive organs, systems and processes are, of course, invaluable, but there is often more to it than this. I take a holistic approach, taking into account the social, emotional and lifestyle context of the couple as well as the pure mechanics of reproduction. The pre-consultation questionnaire provides me with an invaluable tool for assessing this wide range of issues, and also helps many couples to think about their lifestyle and their true aspirations.

Prior to the first consultation, couples who come to my clinic are given a detailed questionnaire, one for women and one for men. This covers:

- the main reason they are seeking a consultation
- fertility history
- contraceptive history
- sexual history
- sexual issues
- general medical history
- family history
- diet and exercise diary
- blood sugar profile
- digestion and elimination profile
- immune profile
- pollution profile
- vitamin and mineral status
- food allergy profile
- details about other hormonal-related conditions that may exist

These questionnaires are long and detailed, to provide, in conjunction with consultation, a full profile on which decisions about the way a couple can choose to proceed can be based.

The questionnaire helps pinpoint areas that may be affecting fertility: factors to do with nutrition and exercise are often highlighted. These may be associated with emotional or lifestyle issues. In this way I try to help couples focus on their situation, so that together we can work out a plan of action. After the initial assessment, we consider what tests, treatments or therapies might be necessary along with the steps a couple need to take for themselves to make conception more possible.

For example, a couple may use cocaine at weekends to relax and chill out. That is their choice, and it is essential that they *do* relax, but the effects are very serious and if they want to conceive a baby they must stop. I try and keep things very simple, with explanations – as you will see in this book – about why change may be necessary. In this way I encourage couples to take responsibility for their own fertility.

It's self-evident that, if you want to improve your likelihood of achieving a successful pregnancy, you have to be willing to make changes. There is often an instinctive reaction against change, but, in truth, the necessary changes are likely to be in areas of your life that you recognize are causing you stress and difficulty. Getting things into perspective for pregnancy is likely to result in a much more balanced, well-managed and satisfactory lifestyle all round – but you need support, advice and encouragement to make this happen.

I see many couples who have already taken steps for themselves along these lines, but this often takes the form of a random blitz of nutritional supplements, complementary therapies, weight-loss regimes, high-protein diets, etc. undertaken without any real knowledge of how these measures will affect their ability to get pregnant. Inevitably, some of these efforts can be unhelpful or even counter-productive.

This problem is not helped by the fragmented nature of available advice. Medical specialists, including obstetricians and gynaecologists, may be engrossed in the mechanics of conception but have little awareness of the patient's emotional or personal situation. Complementary practitioners may have a more holistic view, but are unlikely to be fertility specialists with the appropriate technical knowledge. And nothing in the plethora of highly focused and specialist diets on the shelves of your local bookshop is likely to have been devised with the vital nutritional needs and sensitivities of pregnancy in mind.

Crucial Questions

One way I help couples to understand the need for taking a close look at their lives and finding a way to make the changes necessary to achieve more balance is by asking them to sit down and write out how much time they spend on each area of their lives. You might find this helpful, too, and may want to take a moment to do this for yourself.

In my first session with each couple I always ask a crucial question: How far are you prepared to go to have a baby? Couples just starting out do not realize how important this question is. When you first start trying, you're probably only looking ahead six months or so, and are still very optimistic. The hard thing is that as time goes on there are many things you may have to negotiate: IVF, egg donation, adoption, for example. Where you are on the road now, and the effort you've already spent getting here, will make a difference to the outcome and how far you are prepared to go. Just as you have to be prepared to make changes at the outset, you must also be ready to alter your course as you proceed, as there will be obstacles to encounter and overcome with every success and failure.

This initial, important question makes couples think realistically, often for the first time, about what the quest for a baby might really mean. Sometimes there is a difference of opinion, which can come as a surprise – and is important to discuss. Without agreement on how far a couple want to go to achieve a pregnancy, issues arising from any difference of opinion between partners can lead to tension later on.

There is also a need for flexibility. Minds can be changed, and having opened up the area for discussion it's important for couples to continue to be able to do so.

For those who have reason to suspect they have a problem, there is often little idea of the maze into which the first step to their doctor can take them. Often, in particular if the woman is over 35 and a couple has been trying for a year, there is a tendency to fast-track them into assisted conception – without properly assessing the fertility of either partner.

There is so much that needs to be looked at before assisted conception is even considered, and unless there is significant reason to know that natural conception will be unlikely, this needs to be done *before* catapulting a couple into assisted conception. And again, so often too much focus is put on the woman, when the man very often has the problem. I have seen many valuable months of fertility lost in this way. That said, a lot of couples I see do need assisted conception, but they also need holistic care and support to help ensure that they are physically and emotionally prepared for the process.

Your individual needs

At the end of the first consultation, I draw up a relevant action plan for a couple. Depending on what the consultation has highlighted, this can vary – but it is always specific to the couple. It may include referral for further tests from a gynaecologist and a specialist in male fertility. It is entirely up to a couple how they wish to proceed, but the majority can see that taking a holistic approach is beneficial. Sometimes the action plan is very specific – for example if there is a need to boost the body in preparation for IVF – and sometimes it's more general, where there is a need for fertility awareness and lifestyle changes to improve the chance of conceiving.

I can't stress strongly enough that every couple is a unique combination of needs – both physical and emotional. The way I work is to address that individuality. That said, experience has shown me that when couples have the benefit of a holistic approach – which may encompass medical treatment, nutritional supplementation, relaxation and distressing techniques, detoxifying, acupuncture and massage – the personal outcome for the couple is always positive.

Today's Choices

The difficult choices couples are faced with today are new ones. Years ago, you either had a baby or you didn't. Now the length of time you try can go on almost indefinitely – you start off trying naturally, then perhaps try IVF or egg donation or surrogacy.

Very often I see couples trying for years when certain problems, procedures or decisions could have been reached or ironed out earlier. All this has to be done in the context of a good understanding of a couple's fertility, shared between them and their clinic. It really is a team effort, and one in which the couple are equal partners with the rest of the team.

First Impressions

The process of diagnosis starts the moment a couple walk through my door. I can tell a great deal from the way people walk, their handshake, their posture while seated. For instance, I can tell immediately if a man is inclined to think it is not 'his problem': If he walks in with his head down and arms folded, and avoids eye contact.

As a qualified and practising Five Element Acupuncturist, I use my classical Five Element training to begin assessing each person's constitutional type (see page 223). I look at a person's colouring – not just eye and hair colour, but the texture and hue of his or her skin tone – and I start to build up a picture of an individual's emotional and physical strengths and weaknesses, and in which organs any weakness may be lying. I look at what the general emotion is – worry, anger, grief, fear. Sometimes it's very positive and joyful. I need to understand each person's individual circumstances, and how they are affecting him or her – individually and as part of a couple. I also look for the dynamic between the couple, how vital their relationship is, how close they are, and how they communicate – verbally and non-verbally.

Obviously I take into account that this is an incredibly personal and intimate experience they are sharing with me, which can make many people feel vulnerable. Often they can react defensively, sometimes aggressively, to mask their anxiety. Couples often want me to provide answers, when what I do – and what I hope this book will do for you – is help them find the answers in themselves. Only a full understanding of what you are facing will make it possible for you to make choices, effect any necessary changes and feel positively involved with the process.

I believe that a positive attitude affects the mind and body hugely. The couples I see fall into many categories: those who are starting to try, couples just about to embark on IVF, couples who have had multiple failures, women who have miscarried, couples considering moving on to egg donation, sperm donation, surrogacy or adoption. Help is available to you at every stage of this journey.

If You Are Just Starting Out

Couples in this place tend to be at the end of their twenties or in their early thirties. In many cases the woman has come off the Pill and has no idea what her normal fertility cycle is. It is worth saying here that I don't hold with the belief that a woman shouldn't try to conceive when she first comes off the Pill. The research shows that a woman actually has much *more* chance of conceiving when she first comes off the Pill. Very often, however, women rely on ovulation kits since they don't yet know how to work out their most fertile time. Ovulation kits are fine, but need to be used in conjunction with a knowledge of your cycle. A good biology lesson, as given in Part 1 of this book, removes the element of panic and can put you on the right track. Very often all you need is a fertility awareness session to get you to understand your individual cycle.

At our clinic we also make an assessment of how long a couple have been trying based on age and how often they are having sex, and also give them guidelines for further medical tests they may need alongside the treatments we suggest. At this stage, as far as we know there is no reason why the couple should not get pregnant. Detailed questions can help to pinpoint any lifestyle or nutritional changes that need to be made to enhance fertility, as well as integrating other therapies that might be helpful such as nutrition, acupuncture or hypnotherapy. It might be advantageous to lose some weight, to get your cycle regular using acupuncture, or to assess any emotional issues. Often these quite simple measures make all the difference, and I have seen case after case of straightforward conception in couples who have been trying for some years, and failing, just because of some basic misconceptions that can be readily corrected.

Men are just as important, even in these apparently straightforward cases. If a couple have visited their GP, the man has often had a semen analysis, but seldom understands the implications of the results – not least if they are apparently 'normal'. Not only that, but often semen analyses are done, not in a laboratory, but in a fertility unit and just given a quick check. This is not adequate. A semen analysis should be done under laboratory conditions, assessed by experts and subject to a full analysis, which may include DNA fragmentation (see page 287) and prostatic massage (see page 277) as part of a full sexual health screen. Often a sub-clinical infection with no discernible symptoms is detected that requires antibiotic treatment. Only when there has been an ad-equate analysis, with the proper explanations, is the man likely to take the steps necessary to improve his sperm quality.

Individual fertility cycles

So many couples just don't have sex often enough to get pregnant! However, I don't advocate sex just for the sake of getting pregnant; it should be part of every couple's normal, loving relationship, a way of sharing intimacy and having fun together. That way, sex doesn't become an issue or a chore – where the man thinks the woman is only interested in sex as a means to an end, and not as an expression of her feelings for him. Women, in turn, can become fixated on their fertile time, and only want sex at this time. Prior to this, a couple's rate of sex may have dropped to once week, or a couple of times a month, which may suit them fine – but it's probably not happening enough for a pregnancy to result!

Sex can steadily become mechanical for so many couples; it is so hard for it not to. Many men suffer from 'performance anxiety' around sex if it seems that their partners are only interested in having sex around the time of ovulation. This puts a huge pressure on them. I have heard stories of women emailing their husbands at work, driving to their offices and demanding sex, which inevitably ends in a row and no sex.

If you have been trying for a while, a few basic questions:
- Are you sure you have been having sex at the right time and often enough?
- Are you only interested in sex at the right time of the month and not at any other time?
- Are you still making an effort with your relationship?

Plan ahead; make some of the changes specified in this book before moving on.

If a couple can keep their lines of sexual communication open, and enjoy this aspect of their relationship for its own sake, and not just as a means to pregnancy, then the process will be less stressful all round.

Contrary to popular belief, having sex often does NOT weaken sperm. Research has shown that the more a couple have sex, the more fertility is improved. Here are the figures for women aged 20–30:

Frequency of intercourse per 'monthly cycle'	Delay in months to conception
Once	43 months
Three times a month	15 months
10 times a month	5 months
More than 15 times a month	3½ months

A plan of action

I like couples to leave my clinic with a sense that they have a plan of action, specific to them, and to feel optimistic about it. Together we formulate a four- to six-month action plan, so there is room for a relaxed approach, with the view that the action plan will be reviewed after that. This serves two purposes: it provides both a positive structure and a timescale that takes the pressure off in the short term. This allows a couple to relax, knowing that they have positive steps to take with the opportunity for reviewing the situation in six months' time.

I find that with people in this situation, because the couple have every reason to believe they can get pregnant, they usually do!

If You Have Been Trying for a While

If I could say to couples who have been trying for some time that, by such and such a date, they would be pregnant – they would skip out of my office in delight. But unfortunately there just are no guarantees, and the apparently 'unexplained' causes of infertility are of course the hardest to accept. I often hear women say how difficult they find it when all around them their friends are getting pregnant and having babies. They describe the news of a friend's pregnancy with phrases like 'a knife going through my heart' and find it really difficult to express pleasure or smile at other women's good fortune. Social gatherings become a nightmare, with others asking tactless questions such as, 'When are you starting a family, then?' Nor is it helpful to hear advice such as 'Just relax' or 'Let nature take its course.'

Comments like this may be well meaning, but can result in anger, envy and jealousy, which can in turn lead to feelings of self-hatred. And the stress of it all can lead to quite severe anxiety and depression. Men can be equally affected by these feelings. It's hard on both partners, but women in particular can become obsessed with their monthly cycle, focusing every aspect of their lives on getting pregnant.

Telling a woman not to get obsessive isn't helpful. What *is* helpful is providing a structure for dealing with the reasons behind the obsession, and finding tactics for managing the feelings of frustration, anxiety and sadness that arise.

If couples have been trying for anything from six to 18 months, a lot of emotional and relationship factors start to come into play. For some couples, they find that this shared aim brings them closer together, but often couples can start to feel demoralized and pretty hopeless.

The knock-on effect of this can be detrimental to a couple's sex life. Sex is no longer about intimacy, it has become associated with 'getting pregnant'. Yet, when asked, it can still turn out that the couple are not having sex anything near as often enough to get pregnant. Sex becomes mechanical, with all activity focused on when a woman thinks she's ovulating, so her partner becomes fed up, or afraid that he might not be up to the job when necessary.

This can be further aggravated if a problem has been identified in the man. Coming to see a fertility specialist may be the first time this is openly discussed, and for some men a poor sperm test result makes them feel like a complete failure. The great thing is that there is so much that a man can do to improve the quality and quantity of his sperm production. I would also like to reassure you that, even with a less-than-optimum sperm result, if everything else is going well, conception is still possible. This is important because some couples give up trying at this stage, assuming there is no point. I always encourage couples to keep trying. Many couples go on to conceive, even with a poor sperm result. Nevertheless I do understand that in cases like this it's very hard to be positive.

Sometimes couples become so involved in each other's biological details that all the mystique goes out of the relationship. I saw one couple where the man had taken to examining the cervical secretions in his wife's pants! Another knew every detail of his partner's periods, right down to the consistency of the flow and the amount of blood clots. No wonder some couples' sex lives take a turn for the worse!

A couple's sex life is very important, whatever the circumstances. It is one of the best forms of physical and sensual communication, and can be enormously restorative to a relationship under strain. For those women obsessing about ovulation and insisting on sex there and then, I tell them to stop, throw away the ovulation kits and temperature charts, take a break and put some energy into the relationship, for its own sake. Get romantic, be seductive and take time out together for a walk, a nice meal, a massage, anything shared that can lead to sex within the context of a loving relationship – the same relationship into which you want to bring a baby. The two are not separate, and are paramount to keeping a sense of balance – which is what pregnancy is all about. Creating a family takes energy, a sense of humour, time and love. The other thing about having a good, regular sex life is that it creates a natural high, releasing mood-enhancing endorphins and the bonding hormone oxytocin. I encourage couples to use aromatherapy oils, for massage or in candles – essential oils such as jasmine and ylang ylang stimulate the secretion of endorphins. We all need a little help when times are stressful, so utilize what's available to set the scene and enhance the mood.

The options available

Ultimately you can't control your fertility or when you will get pregnant. But I tell couples that they *can* control the options available to them, and the path they take to get there. It takes a degree of patience to seek out opinions you trust, rather than flit from one fertility plan to another. You need to do the research and then take a step back. Learning to keep a perspective on the situation takes practice – though, naturally enough, many couples find this almost impossible. I find that there is sometimes a tendency for partners to blame one another – even if this is unspoken. This is sometimes not even apparent to the partners themselves, but if I am aware of it I can help diffuse any tension by explaining things and providing a structure for the steps that can be taken.

Another problem can arise when the woman starts to feel she is the one making all the effort. I often find that women drive everything when it comes to trying for a baby: they buy the books, the vitamins, etc., and expect their partner to follow suit. She may try forcing every available vitamin or dietary supplement down her partner's throat, plus enforcing changes in diet and lifestyle, etc. Her partner, meanwhile, may have come to his own conclusions, and very often will only make changes if he has been convinced there is really a problem. Some women make their partners give up absolutely everything, and get fixated about helping their partners make healthy sperm within a precise, limited timeframe. Then if the man lapses, say has a few drinks, the woman gets angry and feels they have to start all over again.

So, for you women: Don't nag. Put time and effort into your relationship and accept that men see it from a different perspective. Be kind to one another. Women can feel extremely angry if they have given up alcohol, or smoking, and their partner hasn't or won't. It feels very unfair, and as if they are making all the sacrifices. Men, for their part, can start to feel very guilty. Obviously, none of this is conducive to success!

For women, with the highs and lows of anticipation during the month, and disappointment if a period arrives, it can be all too easy to get into the blame cycle while forgetting that their partner, too, may be living in dread of a period arriving. Some men start to dread going home, and to feel hopeless about what they can do. Blame can arise from the feeling that 'If only I had done this or hadn't done that' or 'If only he had drunk less or not been on that business trip when I was ovulating …' The permutations are endless.

I know it can be hard, but please try not to start the blame game. Instead, it's important to be kind to each other and remember to share those things that brought you together in the first place.

Keep communicating

It is essential to keep talking. Often things come up in the safety of the consulting room that have been bothering one or other partner. As I've said earlier, trying to get pregnant – especially if it's not happening as expected – is inevitably emotional, and ignoring this can create problems. So I look for opportunities to encourage couples to share their feelings, ideas, and even their resentments! It's much better that these are aired, addressed and resolved than left to fester. I can provide the space for this.

I often recommend couples-counselling for those for whom the situation has become too difficult to deal with. It is far too easy to become estranged through the process of trying to get pregnant. In some cases, I have found that men seem to accept the situation more readily than women. The man may be more relaxed about getting on with life, while his partner may interpret this as a lack of commitment, especially if she is researching on the Internet, seeking out opinions and information, and wanting to focus on getting pregnant almost to the exclusion of everything else. Understandably, many men get fed up, and this can exacerbate the situation still further.

Very often, a few sessions of skilled couples-counselling is all that is needed to bridge the gap, allowing partners to express their feelings and their views, relieve tensions, reduce blame and establish a united platform from which to proceed.

Men need to express how they are feeling, and in the right setting it is amazing what comes out between a couple, especially when a man feels safe about being able to express what he is truly feeling about the situation.

Case History

Linda was 38 and had been trying to get pregnant for two years. She was tearful, angry and upset about her situation. She was on the Internet for up to four hours a day, plus all day at weekends. In the consultation with me, when I asked how it was affecting their relationship, her husband Paul said he had started to dread coming home – Linda would have inevitably found another treatment to pursue, another pill he was going to have to take. He felt completely unable to get through to her; any suggestion he made would get shot down. He felt that Linda was in a total spin; he felt depressed, isolated and fed up of constantly trying to please her. He felt inadequate, and that Linda resented this. His deep, deep concern, which he only felt able to voice in consultation, was that as much as he loved her, he felt that the drive to achieve a pregnancy was becoming destructive for the relationship. Paul had tried to understand Linda's burning desire to have a baby, but he wanted their old life back together where when he came home they had a drink, a chat, a laugh, not him spending time on his own while she was on the Internet.

Linda was able to express that, on her part, she felt panicky that she was running out of time. She felt very stressed and was waking at 4 in the morning and grieving about the child she might never have.

The plan we came up with was to set an absolute limit on Linda's Internet searches and work on getting her internal environment back into balance by doing some yoga and meditation. We did a detox with her to help her lose some weight and we changed the IVF clinic that she was currently attending. Linda got back in contact with me later, to say that our consultation had really been a turning-point. She had not really been aware of the impact her pursuit to have a baby was having on her relationship. Her interpretation of Paul's behaviour was that he wasn't interested in any suggestion she made about treatments, and she felt that he was blocking her at every point. After our consultation she felt she really understood where he was coming from and felt much calmer as a result.

Women in their late thirties/early forties

This age group accounts for a large percentage of the women I see. Often they are career women who have got used to high degrees of control over their environment, and are in uncharted territory when they can't control their own fertility.

Although some come just for a pre-conception 'check', many have been trying for a while. Some have been down the IVF route unsuccessfully; often there is a history of 'unexplained' infertility or recurrent miscarriage, or some anxiety about their fertility cycle. Some couples are taking ovulation-stimulating drugs such as Clomid, or doing intrauterine insemination, and want to improve the chances of conception by supporting and preparing their bodies. Some have been recommended for egg donation without having had a full, clinical work-up or assessment. Very often they have been to only one clinic and were told they have had a poor response and no eggs. Going to another clinic might have meant a better result. In short, there are many factors to consider.

If you have been trying for a while:
- Have you had a diagnosis and have you both been tested?
- How is it affecting you emotionally?
- Are you nagging or resentful of each other?
- Is your relationship starting to suffer?
- Are you losing the balance in your life?
- Are you giving up everything?
- Has your sex life been affected?
- Are you ready to move on to assisted fertility?

The starting-place for these couples has to be an in-depth analysis and discussion with the couple about where they currently feel themselves to be, covering any anxieties or misunderstandings. Without this, there isn't an adequate baseline from which to work. Some couples, especially those who have been round the infertility block a few times, feel that this is unnecessary, as they have already had many medical interviews and tests. In my experience, however, many clinics are not thorough enough when it comes to identifying what the problem might be. Often I find that couples have not even been asked how frequently they have sex! All the medical tests in the world will make no difference if a couple are having sex only twice a month. If the length of a woman's cycle hasn't been worked out properly, any chance of getting the timing of ovulation right is unlikely. As I mentioned earlier, a lot of couples get fast-tracked into assisted conception without a proper assessment. I am sure that this is key to the success we have in helping couples achieve happy, healthy pregnancies.

My Programme

The programme I have devised to help couples always works alongside Western medicine while incorporating complementary therapies and Traditional Chinese Medicine. Looking at the whole picture enables me to come up with an appropriate plan. The main message I try to get across is *keep it simple*. So many couples are running down too many routes with no focus. The initial consultation enables me to look at lifestyle factors and the range of treatments on offer – fertility awareness, nutrition, detox, acupuncture, hypnotherapy, abdominal massage, deep breathing, manual lymphatic drainage (MLD) and counselling. There's more about all of these later in the book. Depending on what suits the couple, usually there are two or three treatments undertaken over a period of four to six weeks, with a review every three months.

The most important thing we offer is support and advice. I believe you can get through anything if you feel supported.

Right from the start, when I first see a couple I stress that they must be flexible in their thinking and not become obsessive. I advise against information overload: endlessly trawling the Internet investigating other people's experiences or solutions may not be relevant, and can even be unhelpful. I recommend trying to keep things in perspective – although many couples feel they have had to give up a lot in order to achieve conception, there is still room to enjoy life as a couple. This should never be forgotten.

I also advise couples to keep in mind that their difficulties with conception, if they arise, are relatively temporary. Actually starting a family may seem like a long haul, but in the greater scheme of things this will represent only a short period in your relationship – it's important to keep this in mind. Long after your fertility problems are resolved, your relationship will still be there – so it's worth nurturing and making time for. A good relationship will also sustain you when things get difficult.

part one
the basics

understanding female fertility

This may sound strange, but many women today have no idea what a normal menstrual cycle is – many of them have been on the Pill for 15 years or more, so this is hardly surprising. Women often feel embarrassed that they don't know everything about their fertility, and this lack of basic knowledge isn't helped by the numerous myths out there about what they should and should not be doing in order to conceive successfully!

I am very fortunate to work alongside Jane Knight, who has done so much to raise awareness for women in this area of fertility. I encourage all women to attend a fertility awareness session, because even if you understand the basics, your cycle is unique to you. At our clinic, the aim is to make it easy to understand when and how ovulation occurs, without getting obsessed about it – which months of 'charting' can do to you. As Jane says:

> An understanding of fertility – fertility awareness – is an important life skill and is every woman's right. My work involves providing fertility-awareness sessions for both men and women. During a consultation I explain how a woman can identify the fertile 'window' during her menstrual cycle. I also help men to understand their own reproductive potential. Couples who understand the key concepts of fertility are

Female Reproductive Organs

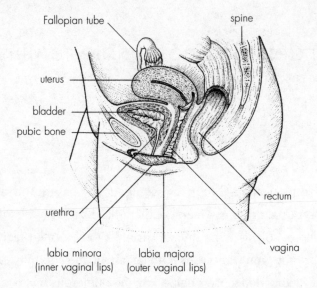

in a much better position to understand how fertility declines with age and how factors may damage, reduce, enhance or optimize fertility.

The primary indicator of fertility for a woman is her *cervical secretions* – because this relates so closely to oestrogen levels and ovulation – so we encourage women to focus on this, alongside ovulation-predictor kits or temperature charting, because it is just as important as good nutrition, relaxation and you and your partner's health in your efforts to conceive.

A Woman's Fertility

At birth, every baby girl is born with a full complement of immature eggs in her ovaries – around 2 million, although only between 300-400 will mature during her lifetime – which sounds as if the whole process should be pretty straightforward. But it is the maturation, release (at ovulation), fertilization and implantation of one of these eggs that results in pregnancy. No new egg cells are produced after you are born, so it's worth thinking about what those egg cells need in order to mature successfully and produce an egg capable of being fertilized. A woman's eggs are her most precious reserve, and need looking after.

Up until puberty, the egg cells lie dormant in the ovaries, waiting for a shift in the hormonal patterns of a girl's body to 'switch on' her fertility. At what age this starts is largely influenced by genetics – if your mother started her periods early, then it's likely you will have done, too. Starting menstrual periods is the marker of the beginning of a woman's fertility, and is known as *menarche.*

In Western countries, the average age of menarche is between 12 and 14, but can be as early as 10 and as late as 16. All are completely normal. Ovulation can occur before the first period, but a girl's early menstrual cycles can be erratic, and often without ovulation. Over the next few months, or sometimes longer, the pattern of cycles settles down to what is normal for that girl, as regular ovulation establishes itself.

If you think back to GCSE biology, you will remember the term 'secondary sex characteristics', which are the outward, visible signs of puberty and the onset of a woman's fertile life. In a woman, increasing levels of FSH (follicle-stimulating hormone) and LH (luteinizing hormone) and the beginnings of oestrogen and progesterone production lead to the development of breast tissue, pubic and underarm hair, and a different distribution of body fat, all of which are designed to create a body capable of nourishing a growing baby, both before and after birth. These changes begin before the first menstrual period occurs, and can happen slowly over a couple of years, or relatively quickly. Again, this depends in part on genetics, and a mother's experience of puberty will give some insight into what her daughter might expect.

Remember how you were warned in your sex education classes at school that sex inevitably led to pregnancy? Remember, too, all the efforts you took in the past not to get pregnant, not to mention all those false alarms? So it may feel a bit of a mystery as to why getting pregnant is now so elusive. This chapter is designed to help you understand your own fertility cycle, and how to work with it to achieve pregnancy.

Understanding Your Own Fertility

With so much misinformation about how, where, why and when, it's always best to start with the basics. Once you are informed and familiar with your own body's fertility indicators, you will feel more confident about managing to get pregnant.

And there is a lot of confusion out there! According to research carried out by Unipath (who produce Persona – the personal hormone-monitoring system), while 92 per cent of women accurately described ovulation, a third of them thought it occurred *during* a period! Out of six European countries covered in the research, the UK women surveyed had the worst knowledge of when their fertile days were: 21 per cent thought they were fertile for more than 21 days a month. And while 72 per cent of women knew that the fertile time was mid-cycle, one-third thought it possible to get pregnant at any time during their cycle.

It is essential to remember that *every woman is different*. Although the basic principles remain the same, what is true of your friend is unlikely to be true of you – from your cycle length to how your body indicates its fertility, to how you react physically and emotionally. This is why it is so useful to understand your own fertility.

Most women seldom think about their fertility, or menstrual cycles, but most women – when they do stop and think about it – are aware of cyclical changes to their skin, appetite, mood – all of which are indicators of their individual cycle.

The Menstrual Cycle

Most of us have learned to live with certain symptoms in our cycle, but it's also important to remember that our fertility cycle is controlled by the pituitary gland, located deep within the brain and influenced by all activity there. Hormones, which are chemical messengers, are primarily controlled by the brain's activity – it's like a constant conversation that occurs between the hormones of the brain and the ovaries, sending messages back and forth (see page 8).

The pituitary gland is often referred to as the 'master gland' of the body, because it secretes at least nine major hormones designed to stimulate the ovaries, adrenals and thyroid, amongst others (including the testes in men), which all have a role to play in fertility. When we are producing the right amount and blend of hormones, we feel fine. When there is an imbalance, these chemical messengers can make us feel pretty lousy. We talk about having 'hormones from hell' when we, as women, feel imbalanced at certain times of the month. PMS is a clear indicator that hormones are out of balance. The hormones are doing their job, and the body is reacting as it should, but because the balance is out, then the effects are negative.

Each of the fertility signals that you observe when you begin to chart your own fertility corresponds to a hormonal process and the presence of hormones in your bloodstream. The hormones oestrogen and progesterone are particularly important, and both affect the body in a number of ways that are easy to note.

The menstrual cycle is a constantly changing hormonal environment, but oestrogen influences the first part of the cycle – up to ovulation – and then progesterone exerts its influence. Some women would probably prefer not to be so influenced by the ups and downs that a cycle brings, but these changing hormonal events will help you to know when your chances of conceiving are best.

Few women have a 28-day cycle, but we can say that the *average* length is around 28 days. For some women their normal cycle can be short (around 25 days) or long (around 35 days). Provided there is a regular pattern, this is normal for you, and you can be relatively sure that ovulation is occurring. It is when cycle length fluctuates from 25 days one month to 30 another, or 42 another, that ovulation is likely to be haphazard, or even non-existent during some cycles.

The fertility, or menstrual, cycle starts on the first day of menstruation or a 'period'. Sometimes on medical forms women are asked to give the date of their 'last menstrual period' or 'LMP' – this would be the date on which you started to bleed.

Oestrogens are the dominant hormones during the first part of the cycle – the time before ovulation, also known as the *follicular phase* (see page 8) – while progesterone takes over during what is known as the *luteal phase* (see page 31) and also during pregnancy, should conception occur. Your cervical secretions are linked to oestrogen secretion, and can give a good indication of the availability of oestrogen.

Menstruation, or a 'period', is the bleeding with which every woman is familiar. It heralds the end of one cycle and the beginning of another. The hormones responsible for the activity of ovulation and womb-preparation effectively 'take a break' at this stage, in order to activate the next cycle. Many women are quite susceptible to the effects of this hormonal switch.

Women often ask me what's 'normal' for a period: how long it should last and how much blood should be lost. The average period lasts for between 3 and 5 days, and the total blood loss is between 30 and 80 ml (6 to 16 teaspoons). However, this is only the average; each woman's experience of her period will be unique to her. Some women seem to have a lot of abdominal cramping (caused by contractions in the womb) when they have a period, or back pain, while others have none. For some, the bleeding happens in a flood at the beginning, while for others it's a slow, continuous bleed.

Hormones and the Phases of Your Cycle

A question I get asked all the time is, 'How do I know if my hormones are balanced?' Hormone balance is such an important part of a woman's fertility, and so easily influenced by poor diet, stress, lack of sleep and environmental factors, that assessing a woman's hormone levels – and addressing any rebalancing that needs to be done to help her achieve optimum fertility – are important aspects of the work I do. And although there are sometimes quite clear indicators of hormone imbalance, often a bit of detective work is needed.

The one major thing that will help balance hormones is a well-balanced lifestyle – which seems to be increasingly difficult for many of us to achieve these days.

A well-balanced lifestyle is important for hormonal balance because all hormone activity is an interplay between different hormones, which are the body's chemical messengers: for example, secretion of fertility hormones will be affected if the body is producing too many stress hormones. Understanding the inter-relationship between all the hormones in the body is the first step towards achieving a positive balance.

Like all hormones, oestrogen and progesterone operate as chemical messengers, in this case controlling the length of a cycle, and ovulation, while also having an impact on other body systems. When in perfect balance, their effects are hardly noticeable, but most women have a degree of hormonal imbalance within the normal range, which makes these hormonal fluctuations more noticeable. Although the effects can vary – not just between women but also from month to month in the same woman – knowing about them and recognizing your own emotional and physical response to them are helpful when you are trying to understand your own cycle.

The Follicular (pre-ovulation) Phase

On Day 1 of the cycle, which is the first day of a period, the brain releases GnRH (gonadotrophin-releasing hormone) from the hypothalamus, which in turn tells the pituitary gland to release FSH (follicle-stimulating hormone). The levels of FSH in the bloodstream build over the next couple of weeks, stimulating follicles in the ovaries to start growing.

The follicle grows and starts to secrete oestrogen from the granulosa cells. It is the rising level of oestrogen that inhibits the secretion of FSH, while also causing ovulation. At this point, LH (luteinizing hormone) is secreted.

This first part of the cycle, the follicular or pre-ovulation phase, can vary in length. This explains why some women have longer cycles than others, and also why their cycles can sometimes be irregular.

The interplay of hormones throughout a woman's fertile life forms the basis of her cycle. Not only do these hormones have a crucial role to play in fertility, they also have other effects on the body, which can be extremely useful when trying to define and assess your own levels of fertility. For example, progesterone has an effect on body temperature (as it's designed to keep a fertilized egg warm in the incubator of the womb), while oestrogen has an effect on cervical secretions, which are so essential to helping achieve pregnancy.

Looking at oestrogen and progesterone individually, and also at how the subtle interplay between them and other hormones affects fertility, is the first step to understanding what is necessary for a pregnancy to happen.

Oestrogen

During the first part of the menstrual cycle, when the levels of oestrogen are rising, endorphins are also released, which are your body's natural painkillers and 'feel-good' hormones, elevating mood. Many women say they feel very energized and creative during this phase.

While oestrogen has an effect on the internal reproductive organs, making the womb receptive to a fertilized egg, bringing the top of the Fallopian tube closer to the ovary and increasing its contractions to help the egg move down towards the womb, it also has other effects.

There are highly specialized cells in the cervix, for example, which produce cervical secretions, and their increased activity is directly caused by increased oestrogen. (The importance of these secretions and their role in conception is crucial, and is explained in more detail on page 18.)

Oestrogen also has an effect on libido, your sex drive. As oestrogen levels rise, so does libido – nature's way of ensuring that sexual intercourse is welcomed close to ovulation. And when an animal is *in oestrus*, i.e. fertile, we refer to them as being 'on heat'. This recognition of a link between oestrogen and heat comes partly from the effect of oestrogen on the blood vessels, causing a degree of dilation and increasing the flow of blood and its heat.

A good blood supply helps the organs of the body function properly, as nutrients are brought to cells and waste products removed. The transportation of oxygen in the blood is also important to developing cells, not least the maturing egg in the ovary. This blood supply also keeps tissues plump and supple, whether in the vagina or the tissues of the face. It is this effect that is lost after the menopause, when the lack of oestrogen causes the thinning of the skin and other tissues.

A good blood flow is beneficial to other organs, too, including the brain. Some women's experience of increased productivity and creativity around ovulation may be explained as their own particular response to oestrogen. On the other hand, for some women this same effect provokes feelings of irritation. It just depends on how your body reacts to and copes with this powerful hormone.

Oestrogen is also essential for maintaining strong bones, as it provides the chemical 'bridge' that allows calcium from the diet to be used by the bones, keeping them dense and reducing porosity.

Oestrogen and Signs of Fertility
The term 'oestrogen' actually refers to a group of hormones that stimulate growth and strengthen tissues. Oestrogen is needed to build up the lining of the uterus so that it can nourish and sustain the fertilized egg, ensuring implantation – a crucial part of conception. When we are talking about fertility, the kind of oestrogen we are referring to is called *oestradiol*. Oestrogen is produced by the developing ovarian follicles and later, in increasing amounts, by the dominant follicle before the egg is released at ovulation.

Oestrogen has many roles:
- It signals the release of LH (luteinizing hormone), needed to trigger ovulation.
- It is needed to build up the endometrium (lining of the womb) so that a fertilized egg can find nourishment and implant successfully.
- It stimulates the production of cervical secretions, which are essential for the sperm to travel through the cervix to the Fallopian tube where an egg may be fertilized.
- It causes the cervix to soften and open, making it easier for the sperm to enter the womb and reach the Fallopian tube for possible fertilization of an egg.

Some of the signs of increased oestrogen levels, such as the amount and quality of cervical secretions, and cervical position, can be easily noticed. These signs offer some of the best indicators of your fertility status. Observing and recording your cervical secretions are vital to assessing fertility, and the optimum time for intercourse, in order to conceive (see page 21).

Factors That Can Affect Oestrogen Production
I often get asked how you can tell if your body is producing enough oestrogen, and what might make you oestrogen-deficient:
- body weight 15–20 per cent below your optimum can cause menstruation to stop, and levels of oestrogen to drop
- an excess of fibre in the diet
- antibiotics – though occasional use is OK
- excessive exercise
- smoking.

Modern women aren't actually *making* more oestrogen; it's just that today's diet and lifestyle encourage higher levels of the hormone in the body. This is in part due to environmental oestrogens, delaying childbirth and breastfeeding, and an over-refined diet. The methods used to clear 'old' oestrogens from the body involve optimum digestive and liver function, which are often compromised by a poor diet and stressful lifestyle. Changing to a low-fat and nutrient-rich diet with adequate (but not too much) fibre can significantly influence the balance of hormones and help to optimize the conditions for getting pregnant.

Equally, an excess of oestrogen can be counter-productive to conception. But take heart: there are ways round these issues – we'll be taking a look at them in the Nutrition chapter.

The Ovulation Phase

The rising oestrogen level makes the hypothalamus reduce the secretion of GnRH and FSH. As the FSH decreases, oestrogen levels from the maturing follicle rise abruptly. Only then will the pituitary gland secrete LH (luteinizing hormone), which allows just one mature follicle to release an egg – ovulation.

The Magnificent Egg

The ovum, or egg, is the largest cell in the body – 550 times bigger than the sperm. As it matures within its fluid-filled follicle prior to ovulation, it needs a lot of energy, which is supplied by the granulosa cells (specialized cells in the ovary). These cells have two functions: to secrete oestrogen (to help the egg mature) and to nourish and feed the egg as it grows.

The maturing egg is now suspended in a fluid-filled cavity (sometimes referred to as the *graafian* follicle, after the scientist who first discovered it). This follicle measures about 18–23mm just prior to ovulation, and when ovulation – the release of the egg – occurs, the follicle bursts and the mature egg is released into the Fallopian tube.

There are an estimated 7 million granulosa cells packed around an egg, greatly increasing the availability of energy. When the egg is eventually released, it takes with it a mass of these cells, giving it a 'sunburst' appearance. These cells also serve to protect and nourish the egg on its journey, and will provide a barrier against all but the one sperm that will fertilize it.

The hormonal stimulus for ovulation is the rise of oestrogen, and the primary factor that determines when you will ovulate is the level of oestrogen getting to a certain threshold, which creates a surge in luteinizing hormone (LH), responsible for the rupture of the follicle and release of the egg. So anything that depletes oestrogen will keep it from reaching the necessary level, and ovulation will not take place.

Ovulation also won't occur unless the optimum level of oestrogen is maintained for the correct length of time. The timing of ovulation is quite exact, occurring about 36 hours after the surge in LH. Only a mature egg, once fertilized, will result in conception. Immature eggs are unlikely to be capable of being fertilized, and even if they are they tend to produce an abnormal embryo that won't implant or develop properly, resulting in an early miscarriage (before 12 weeks). So it's very important that the level of oestrogen produced accurately reflects the egg's maturity. It's a delicate feedback process, and the timing is crucial. A mature egg is necessary for fertilization because only then will it have chromosomes at the right stage for further development, allowing one sperm in and blocking the rest, and ensuring that the egg and sperm fuse properly.

At the same time, just before ovulation the follicle generates a rapid rise in the hormone progesterone. The rise in progesterone also keeps the FSH secretion going just long enough to allow full maturation of the follicle. As the hypothalamus is shutting down on FSH secretion, it is releasing prostaglandins to the follicle just before it ruptures. It is thought that these prostaglandins may help to expel the egg by breaking down the follicle wall.

Once the egg is released, the resulting cavity and the remaining granulosa cells start to produce more progesterone. These cells also stain the ruptured follicle an orangey-yellow colour, giving rise to the name *corpus luteum*, from the Latin for 'yellow body'.

The egg is at its most susceptible to nutrient deficiency during this phase of the menstrual cycle, leading up to ovulation where the egg is maturing, and during early embryonic life (the first 30 days after conception). Research shows that a 70 per cent increase in sensitivity to toxins, alcohol and smoke occurs between 11.30 a.m. and 7 p.m. on the day preceding ovulation. In the five days prior to ovulation a good diet and as few toxins as possible are particularly important for achieving pregnancy. Also, it is not wise to drink heavily during this phase of your cycle. If the diet is too low in proteins, for example, too few eggs may ripen, while a vitamin B1 deficiency can inhibit ovulation. Because it can be difficult to gauge exactly when ovulation occurs, however, it is always wise to maintain good nutrition *throughout* your cycle.

Lifespan of the Egg

Having managed to ovulate a mature, functioning egg and, with all other things working to advantage, the lifespan of the egg is only estimated to be around 8 to 12 hours. This is further complicated by the difficulty in knowing exactly when ovulation occurs. For example, if you ovulate at 3 a.m. but don't have intercourse until the following evening, chances are that the egg is no longer capable of being fertilized. Now, I wouldn't want any woman reading this to start lying awake at night worrying that she might be ovulating then and there – this won't help you or your partner in the long run! – but this is why regular and frequent sex is an essential feature of successful conception. Keep in mind that sperm deposited in a woman's vagina stay alive, on average, for between two and three days (and in some cases for up to a week), so if you are having sex every day or every couple of days around the most fertile time of your cycle, the chances of conception are increased dramatically. Research shows that most pregnancies occur within a 'fertile window' of six days before ovulation and one day after. If there are live, potent sperm in the Fallopian tubes when ovulation occurs, then conception is much more likely than if sex occurs sometime after ovulation.

Why Cycle Length Matters

The length of the menstrual cycle is measured from the first day of menstruation (first day of fresh bleeding) up to the day before the next period starts. The time you are fertile will vary according to the length of your cycle. The time from ovulation to the next period is likely to be constant – approximately 10 to 16 days – whereas the time before you ovulate can be more variable.

The fertile time in a woman's cycle is identified by two different approaches:

1. by looking at the length of your cycle and making calculations based on observing your secretions (see page 22)

2. by a combination of recording your temperature and knowing the position of your cervix (see page 22) – though I don't usually encourage women to use these measures, as trying to do so can be confusing and stressful.

Understanding that the post-ovulation phase remains constant at around 14 days, while the pre-ovulation phase is the one that's variable, is essential because this will help you to work out, roughly, when you are ovulating. Once you have a rough idea of what's normal for you, working out the other indicators of fertility becomes easier.

Only if a woman's cycle is a regular 28 days does she ovulate mid-cycle, around day 14. If her regular cycle is 25 days, then ovulation occurs around day 11; a cycle of 35 days means ovulation around day 21; and for a very long cycle of 42 days, ovulation occurs around day 28.

Many women mistakenly believe that ovulation occurs 'mid-cycle', then wonder why they are getting their calculations wrong. Everywhere this myth continues to be perpetuated, and it can really hamper couples' attempts to conceive. For example, if you thought the *middle* of your 35-day cycle was when you were ovulating, you'd think this was day 17 – when in fact, it's day 21 – and would thereby make a crucial error when it came to timing sexual intercourse to coincide with your fertile time.

If you don't have an understanding of this basic information about the two phases of the menstrual cycle, all the other indicators of fertility you are trying to evaluate just won't 'add up'.

Case History: Christine

Christine, who was 34, had had one child with IVF. Two further attempts at IVF had been unsuccessful. She came along to our clinic to see what she could do to improve her chances. Having looked through her questionnaire, apart from the fact that she was tired from coping with a toddler, and also a little bit underweight, there were no obvious lifestyle factors that might be affecting her chances. I went back to basics with her and asked about her cycles and sex, and suggested that, as she had irregular cycles, a session of fertility awareness would benefit her. I could tell she thought that this would be a total waste of time, as she'd been told that she wasn't ovulating.

'How do you know you don't ovulate?' I asked. She said that when she used the ovulation-predictor kits (see below), nothing happened. When I asked about her cervical secretions, she said she didn't have any. Then I started to ask about her periods and how long her bleed lasted. Her bleed lasted 7 days, and on the 8th and 9th days there was what she thought was mucus but mixed with the blood; she also thought that this was part of her bleed. Her cycles were quite varied – between 28 and 38 days – so by her calculations if anything were going to happen it wouldn't be on the 8th or 9th day of her period; it would be much later in the cycle. She was wrong about this.

She went on to conceive naturally a month later.

I could write about many more cases like this, of women who have had IVF when they have never even been offered the most basic kind of help with understanding their fertility.

Ovulation Predictor Kits

Luteinizing hormone can be measured by ovulation-predictor kits, which use chemicals to identify the presence of LH in your urine. LH is not released all at once, but rises and falls for 24 to 48 hours. The LH rise usually begins in the early morning while you are sleeping; it appears in your urine about 4 to 6 hours later. For this reason, first-morning urine may not give the best result. It is important to follow the instructions on the kit for optimum results.

If you are able to recognize the pattern of your cervical secretions, ovulation-predictor kits have little value except to reassure you. You may just want to use them to cross-check your other signs of impending ovulation. If you have irregular cycles or multiple patches of fertile cervical secretions before ovulation, however, ovulation kits can be helpful.

I think ovulation-predictor kits are fine – so long as they're used in conjunction with examining your cervical secretions (see below). They can also encourage women to have sex only when the predictor kit indicates – therefore missing out on opportunities for sex during the preceding five days, which is essential to maximize the chances of conception.

There is absolutely no point rushing out and buying an ovulation-predictor kit if you don't have at least a rough idea of your cycle. I see women who have got into a real muddle using them, and have often convinced themselves that they're not ovulating because, without any idea of what their normal cycle is, they've used the kit at the wrong time.

Once you know your own, individual cycle, the kit can help confirm when ovulation is coming up – but by then you will be so confident of reading your own body's fertility indicators that you won't need it!

Cervical Secretions

Your secretions are your fertility. It is my hope that all women trying for a baby get to know and focus on this. If you take only one thing from this chapter, take this: recognizing the range of and changes to your secretions is key to understanding your fertility, because they are so closely linked to oestrogen levels.

Cervical secretions are produced continuously by the glands lining the cervix, and provide a slightly acidic barrier during the infertile phase of your menstrual cycle, protecting against any bacteria or germs that can enter the body via the vagina.

These secretions are influenced by the changing hormones of your cycle, as we have seen, and provide the most useful indicator of hormonal activity. Highly fertile secretions, which tend to resemble raw egg white, are stimulated by peak oestrogen levels, and not only indicate that ovulation is imminent, but also provide channels for the sperm to swim along and an optimum environment for sperm. Influenced by oestrogen, the secretions at this time are also more alkaline, protecting the sperm from the normal acidity of the vagina.

For women who have spent a long time on the Pill, cervical secretions and the way they change during a cycle can be something of a mystery. Coming up to ovulation, cervical secretions become more obvious, but only by looking at and feeling them can a woman be really sure of what stage in her cycle she is at.

Oestrogen and cervical secretions

The easiest way to assess the presence and quantity of oestrogen in your bloodstream, and gain clues about your fertility status, is to check your cervical secretions throughout your cycle.

Increased production of oestrogen, as your body prepares for ovulation, stimulates the cells of the cervix to produce more secretions, which creates an increasingly wet and slippery feeling around the vagina as you approach ovulation. While your cervical secretion pattern may vary from cycle to cycle, a typical cervical secretion pattern over the course of a menstrual cycle will look like this:

- Day 1 of your cycle is marked by bleeding, which may continue for between 3 and 5 days, depending on what is normal for you.
- Immediately following the end of a period, cervical secretions aren't produced in any noticeable quantities and the vagina can be described as quite dry.
- After a couple of days, you may notice a creamy-white secretion which has no odour and produces no discomfort. It may leave a bit of a mark on undergarments.
- This creamy-white secretion then becomes a little thinner and whiter, and increases a little in quantity. Some women have described this as being similar in colour and consistency to moisturizing lotion.
- Over the next couple of days these secretions change quite dramatically, becoming increasingly more clear and 'elastic'.
- Just prior to ovulation, cervical secretions become completely clear, exceedingly 'stretchy' and can be described as resembling raw egg white. This is the peak time for cervical-secretion production, and with good reason: for sperm to reach an egg they need to be able to swim upwards, and through a lubricated channel that allows this. In addition, when looked at under a microscope, these cervical secretions appear to have channels within them, assisting the sperm even further. Not all women notice the elasticity or stretchiness of these highly fertile secretions, but they may simply be aware of an increased wetness. Some women even describe this as feeling as if they have wet themselves. This may be because this type of secretion is produced in small 'pulses' from the top of the cervix.

- Almost immediately following ovulation, the cervical secretions stop being clear and stretchy, and revert back to a thicker creamy secretion, which can become quite 'blobby' over the next few days. This is the progesterone effect. It creates a bit of a seal to the cervix (neck of the womb), designed to prevent any foreign bodies – from sperm to bacteria – ascending the womb. It also makes the vagina more acidic and hostile to sperm.
- Over the next couple of weeks, leading up to the next period, cervical secretions become minimal again, producing just enough to keep the vaginal canal moist and protected.

When you first attempt to identify and interpret your own cervical secretion changes, it's worth being aware of the factors that can make this difficult. Wash as normal, using soap and water and rinsing well, but avoid the use of vaginal deodorants, talcum powder or lubricating jellies. Wear all-cotton underwear, and avoid absorbent pads, thongs, G-strings or nylon tights – stockings are better!

Television adverts for panty-liners have broached the subject of cervical secretions, although not overtly, preferring to refer to those 'in-between days' when you need some protection. Certainly, for some women, the secretion of cervical mucus can be copious and very watery at times. However, I don't recommend the use of panty liners, as they can be very drying and too absorbent, so many women miss their fertile secretions. Better to bring a spare pair of pants to change into during the day if necessary.

In summary, the general pattern is for cervical secretions to change throughout the menstrual cycle, increasing in quantity and becoming more clear (transparent) and stretchy as you get closer to ovulation. Noticing and recording these changes for a few months will help you recognize your individual fertility pattern. In the most common pattern, as mentioned, cervical secretions start out dry (just after your period) and then get sticky, then creamy, then wet and watery, becoming most like raw egg white as you get closer to ovulation. You may, though, get different types of cervical secretions on the same day. Always record your most fertile cervical secretions to make sure that you do not miss a potentially fertile day.

How to check for cervical secretions

Avoid checking your cervical secretions just before or after intercourse, as arousal and seminal fluids will skew your observations. The best way to check your cervical secretions is to make observations whenever you go to the bathroom. After you wipe, note what, if anything, you find on the bathroom tissue. This will soon become second nature and you will find yourself noticing your cervical secretions every time you use the toilet. You can also use clean fingers to check for cervical secretions, and you may also notice some in your underwear.

What to Look For
- Does your vagina feel wet or dry?
- Are there any secretions on the bathroom tissue?
- How do they look?
- What colour are they?
- What consistency are they?
- How much is there?
- How do they feel when you touch them?
- Can you stretch them between your thumb and index finger?

Exercise, and having a bowel movement, will push cervical secretions to the vaginal opening, making observation easier. You may even find that the best time to check is after a bowel movement.

Position of the Cervix

Just a quick word about this: Women are stressed enough trying to conceive without trying to find out what position their cervix is in – and trying to check this might also interfere with or obscure any cervical secretions you have got! I don't believe that the position of your cervix is a useful enough indicator for women trying to have a baby.

Keeping a record

Always record your most fertile type of cervical secretions, even if you notice more than one type on any given day or even if it is scant. This is so that you won't miss a potentially fertile day and so that you have a consistent record of your cervical secretions from cycle to cycle.

Immediately after a period you may notice one or more dry days – when no secretions can be seen or felt (these days are not likely to be fertile). As soon as the secretions start, this means that the cervix is preparing to accept sperm and you are into the start of your fertile time. At first the secretions will feel slightly sticky and be white or creamy in colour, then they'll gradually change to become cloudy and wetter, then more transparent and sometimes quite slippery and stretchy – the highly fertile sperm-friendly secretions. After ovulation the secretions change back to being thicker, more sticky and white again, then back to dry again in the run-up to your next period. As a quick 'rule of thumb', if you feel wet – have lots of sex!

FERTILITY AWARENESS CHART – planning pregnancy

Chart no.	Date: May 2002																																								
	Day	W	T	F	S	S	M	T	W	T	F	S	S	M	T	W	T	F	S	S	M	T	W	T	F	S	S	M	T	W	T	F	S	S	M	T	W	T	F	S	S
	Ovulation predictor kits												LH																												
Cervical secretions	Wet, slippery, transparent, stretchy											■																													
	Moist, white, cloudy, sticky								■					■																											
	Dry-No secretions seen or felt						■									■	■	■	■	■	■	■	■	■	■	■															
	Period		■	■	■																						■														
	Day of Cycle – Circle intercourse	1	2	3	4	5	6	⑦	8	⑨	10	⑪	⑫	⑬	⑭	15	16	17	⑱	19	20	㉑	22	23	㉔	25	26	27	28	29	30	31	32	33	34	35	36	37	38	39	40

Example Chart

Factors that can influence your pattern of secretions

Some factors that can influence the quality and quantity of cervical secretions that you produce may be a result of hormonal factors, while others may be related to lifestyle or medications you are taking. If any of these applies to your case, make a note. If you are using a fertility-awareness chart there is usually a special section where you can do this. This way you can see at a glance if there were any special circumstances that may have had a bearing on your cervical secretions.

Factors that can have an impact on cervical secretion patterns include:

- medications such as antihistamines and diuretics
- fertility medication such as Clomid (ask your doctor)
- tranquillizers
- antibiotics
- expectorants – as found in cough medicines
- herbs (ask your doctor before taking herbs while trying to conceive)
- vitamins such as vitamin C (over 1,000mg a day), as this may have an anti-histamine effect, reducing cervical secretions and making them more acidic
- vaginal or sexually-transmitted infection (ask your doctor if you think this is a possibility)
- delayed ovulation (can cause an interrupted pattern of secretions)
- vaginal douching (not recommended)
- being overweight
- arousal fluid (can be mistaken for raw egg white cervical secretions)
- semen residue (can be mistaken for raw egg white cervical secretions)
- lubricants (not recommended when trying to conceive, as they can be hostile to sperm)
- breastfeeding – high levels of prolactin suppress oestrogen secretion
- decreased ovarian function – for example in the years approaching the menopause

- after you've stopped taking the Pill – a normal cycle may not have had a chance to re-establish itself. (Remember, though, that it's still a good idea to have regular sex even if you've just come off the Pill!)

If you notice anything that concerns you about your cervical secretions, for example if they are smelly or causing you discomfort or itchiness, or if you are bleeding or spotting, see your doctor. Any infection must be treated (for more about routine tests for infections, see the Fertility Work-up chapter).

If you have questions about how to observe and interpret your cervical secretions, or if you have specific concerns about your own experience, then it's well worth finding a fertility awareness teacher (see Useful Contacts, page 358).

No Raw Egg White Secretions

If you do not see any cervical secretions that resemble raw egg white, the first thing to do is to check out how you are observing this, especially if you are new to it (see page 21). If you are sure you are checking properly, but your cycles are irregular, you may not be ovulating every time. If your cycles are regular, then your secretions may have been affected by one of the factors outlined above. As long as you are having sex every other day or so, then the absence of an obvious indication of imminent ovulation is not something you should worry about too much.

Fertile Cervical Secretions after Ovulation

Some women notice what seems like highly fertile cervical secretions (wetter, transparent and stretchy) around the time they are expecting their period. This is because towards the end of the cycle there are some hormonal fluctuations between oestrogen and progesterone. As the progesterone level falls (due to the degeneration of the corpus luteum), the secretions appear more oestrogen-dominant. These secretions, how-ever, should *not* be interpreted as a sign of fertility.

Predicting Ovulation

Predicting ovulation is not a precise science, but familiarity with your cervical secretions makes it a whole lot easier. The general advice is always to have lots of sex, rather than limiting it to a specific time – but when the pressure is on to conceive, sex can lose some of its sponta-neity, which makes knowing the most fertile time of your cycle useful.

Try and keep some perspective about this, and don't restrict sex to an exercise in conception – try and make sure you and your partner enjoy it for its own sake, too, and as a way to express your loving feelings for each other.

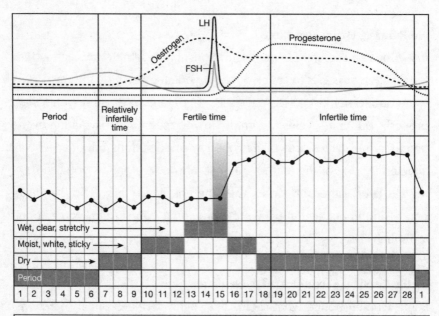

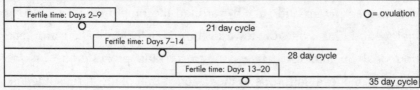

© Dr Cecilia Pyper and Jane Knight 1999 in collaboration with Fertility UK.

Cervical Secretions and Semen

If you find that you have more watery or raw egg white days than you would expect and that these often follow days or nights when you've had intercourse, then you may be mistaking seminal fluid for cervical secretions. They are quite similar, but remember that fertile cervical secretions are clear, stretchy and shiny. They can stretch a couple of inches without breaking. Semen may be more whitish and will break when pulled. Generally if you have had sex the night before, by lunchtime the following day there should be no trace of semen and you should be able to concentrate on your secretions.

Many women continue to experience a degree of cervical secretion after ovulation (necessary to keep the vagina moist and healthy) because the corpus luteum produces small amounts of oestrogen along with larger amounts of progesterone. However, this is no indicator of fertility: once ovulation has occurred for a cycle, it won't occur again until the next one.

When you first start to take note of your secretions, they may be erratic and won't follow the usual pattern of dry, sticky and white→clear and wet→sticky, white and dry again. Stick with it; it may take a while to work out.

Increasing cervical secretions

Evening Primrose oil (EPO) can play a role in the production of quality cervical secretions. EPO is an essential fatty acid (EFA) that contains gamma-linolenic acid (GLA), which is converted to a hormone-like substance called prostaglandin E1. EPO helps the body to produce raw egg white cervical secretions.

The recommendation is to take a supplement of EPO only during the first, pre-ovulatory time of the cycle, from menstruation to ovulation. This is because of the slight risk that EPO can cause uterine contractions, which you would want to avoid after ovulation. The recommended dose for the time between your period and ovulation should be 1,500 to 3,000mg per day (see Nutrition chapter for more details).

It may take a month or two to build up and produce the results you are looking for. If you are keeping a record of your fertility signs over the months, this will help you identify the first part of your cycle, prior to ovulation, when taking this supplement is advised. You will also know when you have ovulated, so you'll know when to stop taking the EPO.

However, if you have had a diagnosis of high oestrogen levels, you will not know when you have ovulated and taking EPO will not be advised because of its oestrogenic properties. Far better, in this case, to visit a nutritionist and get an individually-tailored programme.

Other Ways to Increase Secretions
- Drinking plenty of water will increase your internal fluid balance and make any bodily secretion more fluid.
- Avoiding antihistamines, which reduce mucus secretions.
- Avoid high doses of vitamin C (more than 1,000mg per day).

Does Robitussin Really Work?
In chat rooms across the Internet, hundreds of women swear by taking 2 tablespoons of cough medicine that contains guaifenesin as the only active ingredient before ovulation. (Guaifenesin works as an expectorant to increase the liquidity of mucus production in the lungs, and elsewhere, to make coughing up phlegm easier.) It is believed that this makes cervical mucus more liquid and hospitable to sperm. While this may work in principle – and anecdotal evidence is eagerly repeated – there is little scientific evidence to back it up, although one 20-year-old study does indicate that it can be helpful in thinning out cervical mucus.

If you are going to take it, you would want to do so about five days before and including the day of ovulation. However, when you are trying to conceive it's worth thinking about the effects of any medication that you take, even those bought over the counter. There are some women who have allergic reactions to guaifenesin, although it is generally considered safe. Make sure there are no other ingredients in the cough mixture that could be harmful – check with your pharmacist.

Progesterone and Your Cycle

While oestrogen dominates the first phase of your cycle, progesterone dominates your second, post-ovulatory or luteal phase of your cycle. Before ovulation, progesterone is present only in small amounts. After ovulation, progesterone, produced by the corpus luteum, is present in higher amounts.

Progesterone has many roles:

- It makes the lining of your uterus soft and spongy, with increased blood flow, so that a fertilized egg can latch on to it and implant.
- It is needed to support and continue a pregnancy by ensuring that the lining of the womb remains intact and a woman doesn't have a period.
- It also causes your Basal Body Temperature (BBT) to rise after ovulation so that it is measurable with a BBT thermometer.

Although some women choose to record their waking temperature, many of the women I see get so stressed out by this method that I do not normally recommend it. Nor is this method recommended by new NHS guidelines – for three reasons:

1. Progesterone causes a rise in BBT (that is, waking temperature – your temperature after you have been resting for at least three hours and before you get out of bed).

2. Your temperature does not rise until AFTER ovulation – by which time it is too late to try to conceive.
3. It can be very stressful having a daily reminder when you first wake up that you are not pregnant yet.

As I said earlier, generally I would not advise women to record their temperature. There may be an appropriate role for taking your temperature if you have been advised by a trained fertility awareness practitioner that this would be beneficial – for example to provide a more objective marker and to determine the length of the luteal phase of your cycle. Otherwise – don't worry about it.

Having said this, taking their temperature does give some women reassurance that they are ovulating. Trying this for a month when you are first trying to conceive will do no harm, but not month in, month out – it causes too much stress. Many factors affect your temperature – a low-grade fever, alcohol, fewer than three hours' sleep, air travel and electric blankets – so it's really not the best indicator.

Because progesterone is the hormone designed to prepare the body for pregnancy, birth and breastfeeding, its effects are linked to these processes. Breasts tend to swell a little under its influence, and can become tender for many women during the second phase of their cycle (and during early pregnancy, if it occurs).

Progesterone also has an effect on muscles in the body, for example in the gut, making digestion less efficient. This can make some women more prone to constipation (another common problem for many women during pregnancy).

In addition, the progesterone effect on smooth muscle affects the ligaments, which soften. This is in preparation for labour, when the ligaments of the pelvis have to soften for the bones to 'give' a little during birth. Although this is not so extreme as during pregnancy, some women find they are more susceptible to minor injuries after ovulation, when progesterone levels are raised.

Some women whose blood pressure is naturally low may find these combined effects of progesterone can cause them to feel a bit faint, or more tired, in the run-up to their period. Ensuring an adequate intake of fluids, while avoiding those with diuretic effects like colas, coffee and large quantities of tea, can help with this.

Luteal or Post-ovulatory Phase

Progesterone is the hormone that keeps the endometrium, or lining of the womb, in place. It keeps it thick and ensures a continuing blood supply – just in case a fertilized egg needs to implant. If implantation does occur, the production of progesterone from the ovary continues until around 12 weeks, when the placenta is sufficiently developed to take over production for the rest of the pregnancy. If there is no implantation, the body responds by reducing its levels of progesterone, and a period occurs – when the thick, blood-rich lining of the womb is discarded.

Progesterone Deficiency

Progesterone deficiency is the most common hormonal deficiency in women of all ages. Many women are already familiar with the symptoms of a degree of progesterone deficiency, which may or may not affect their fertility. These symptoms include painful or lumpy breasts, cyclical headaches, anxiety and irritability, insomnia and sleep problems, unexplained weight gain, recognizable PMS, dysfunctional patterns of bleeding during a cycle, and finally, impaired fertility.

The causes of progesterone deficiency are often linked to imbalances of other hormones, and the effect of these. For example, if ovulation fails, no progesterone is produced in the luteal phase. There may also be defects during the luteal phase – either the corpus luteum fails to produce enough progesterone, doesn't produce it for long enough, or the luteal phase is too short (fewer than 10 days). In addition, in some cases the follicle develops but doesn't rupture and expel the egg, so too little progesterone is produced. Finally, the messages from the hypothalamus and pituitary gland may be faulty – there is faulty FSH secretion, inappropriate surges of LH or excessive prolactin.

Having identified a progesterone deficiency, there are a number of solutions:

- natural progesterone (should only be used under proper medical supervision)
- vitamin and mineral deficiencies can be remedied (supplements for low progesterone include vitamin B6, vitamin E, evening primrose oil and magnesium)
- herbs such as Vitex Agnus Castus, prescribed by a medical herbalist, can help regulate ovulation
- causes of stress can be identified and removed
- excessive exercise can be reduced
- low body weight can be increased.

A Time to Reflect

I encourage women to see their period as a time of contemplation and renewal, and to see the process of bleeding as cleansing. Our modern lifestyles encourage women to disregard how they feel during their period, advocating the use of tampons and treating this phase of the cycle just the same as any other. I encourage women to use this time to reflect and to recharge their emotional and physical batteries. It is perfectly natural that very often women find themselves not wanting to socialize during this time, preferring to be quiet and reflective.

What is useful for me when I am working with a woman is to know what a 'normal' period is for her, so I can see how this relates to the rest of her cycle.

In Traditional Chinese Medicine (TCM), much more attention is paid to a woman's period than in Western medicine. The length of a period and the colour, amount and quality of the blood flow are all considered, alongside other information and observations (see page 217). In my work I use the principles of Five Element Acupuncture, a feature of TCM that I find very useful in assessing each woman and her individual concerns or problems.

Period pains, if severe, can be indicative of the sort of hormonal upsets that suggest problems in the menstrual cycle. In TCM it isn't considered normal to have painful periods; this is seen as an indication that some sort of hormonal rebalancing is needed. In the West, many women accept that their periods are painful, and take large quantities of painkillers in order to function, without realizing that these drugs can be detrimental to their fertility (see page 172). TCM, and acupuncture in particular, along with abdominal massage (see page 229) can all help in alleviating not just the pain but also the cause of it. This is a much better alternative to swallowing lots of painkillers, some of which are quite strong and anti-spasmodic, which can in turn interfere with the menstrual cycle. I also believe that it's far better for women to use nutritional means to deal with painful periods. Taking an EFA (essential fatty acid) supplement, and one that contains evening primrose oil (GLA) can help normalize the hormones called *prostaglandins*. Period pains can be an indicator that prostaglandins are being over-produced, which can, in turn, have an impact on your overall hormonal cycle and may affect your fertility.

Women with severe period cramps often show a depletion in the mineral magnesium, for example, and taking a supplement of this – which helps with muscular tension – can help to alleviate the pain.

For women trying to conceive, the arrival of their period can be a time of sadness as it means conception hasn't been successful that month. There is no question that the emotional response to this can be quite profound, and it can also be exacerbated by hormonal changes. However, the menstrual period can also be seen as a sign for optimism, as it can be used for contemplation, renewal and preparation – physically and emotionally – for the next cycle and another opportunity – with increasing knowledge – for conception.

I think it's better for women to use pads rather than tampons during their period, especially if they suffer from endometriosis. I realize that this isn't always practical, especially if the bleeding is very heavy, but women should be aware that tampons can be very drying to the vagina, absorbing normal vaginal moisture. If you are going to use tampons, opt for those made with organic, non-bleached cotton, and use pads on lighter days. TCM also recommends keeping the abdominal area warm, either with direct heat (from a hot water bottle, for example) or through warming, nourishing foods – especially when there is discomfort during a period.

Keeping a Diary

First of all, without making a daily note of where you are in your cycle, it's hard to gauge your individual pattern of fertility, either for yourself or for a health professional. Many of the women I see keep note of the length of their periods. Knowing roughly the length of your previous six cycles, the length of the shortest and of the longest can be a big help in identifying your fertile time: your shortest cycle minus 20 gives you your first fertile day, and your longest cycle minus 10 gives you your last fertile day.

Your diary should record the following:

- First day of your period (Day 1 of your cycle).
- Signs of cervical mucus (particularly noting the very fertile clear, wet, stretchy secretions).
- Lifestyle notes (evenings out, alcohol intake, stress at work, travel, holidays, etc.)
- Use of any medicines – such as painkillers for headaches, antihistamines, antibiotics, etc.
- Occasions of full sexual intercourse.
- Libido.
- Physical feelings – abdominal cramps, headache, energy levels, breast tenderness, etc.
- Emotions – moods, happiness, irritation, etc.

Most women need to observe their secretions for about three cycles before they feel confident about recognizing changes. Do bear in mind that keeping a diary is designed to provide you with an overview of your cycle, not a foolproof means to conception. It is all too easy to get obsessive about these things – try to keep a sense of perspective.

One of the reasons keeping a diary is so useful is that it is only possible to evaluate your cycle length retrospectively. It's only after keeping a note of several cycles that any sort of recognizable pattern will begin to emerge. If you have been on the contraceptive pill, or have no idea of what your cycle length might actually be, then keeping a diary noting down this information before trying to get pregnant can be enormously helpful and quite revealing. It also provides you with an objective record of events, which can be equally helpful in identifying problems such as a fluctuating cycle length, inadequate frequency of sexual intercourse, use of medication, etc.

Even though fertility awareness seems to involve a lot of information, as you become more aware of what is happening during your cycle, it soon becomes second nature. What is important, however, is to remain aware without becoming obsessive. When all's said and done, the single thing that is most likely to improve your chances of conception is having lots of sex, not just sex at specific times. If you can do this without focusing solely on procreation, but keeping the pleasure in mind, it can only be beneficial for both you and your partner.

Questions and Answers

What if I have a brown discharge for a few days before my period starts? Does this count as Day 1?
No, Day 1 is the first full flow of blood, the first day of red bleeding.

I have just come off the Pill and want to get my system cleaned up before starting to try for a baby.
Don't, because research shows that you are more fertile in the first couple of months that you come off the Pill. Getting pregnant can become harder in following months.

Most women get pregnant very quickly after stopping the Pill – in fact, some fertility clinics put women on the Pill to get the 'rebound' fertility effect. With newer lower-dose pills, there is no reason to wait for the Pill hormones to get out of your body. There are no adverse effects shown if you get pregnant immediately after stopping the Pill (or other hormonal methods of contraception).

Will it take time to get pregnant following taking the Pill?
Some women get pregnant straight away, while for others it takes time to get their cycles back on a regular basis. It can be harder for some women to conceive after stopping the Pill – particularly if they are over 30 years old and have never had a child. So planning ahead is useful.

You could also check your rubella status (by having a simple blood test) while still on the Pill, because if you need to have a vaccination it is essential that you are not pregnant.

One of the disadvantages of the very effective contraceptive Pill, on which many of us rely to control our fertility, is that it wipes out a woman's individual menstrual cycle, which is of course its aim. The doses of hormones given to achieve this have to be large enough to over-ride a woman's own hormones, and this tends to blanket any normal fluctuation and effects a woman might recognize.

Coming off the Pill to get pregnant means also getting back in touch with those signs and symptoms of fertility, some of which might not be welcome if the Pill was prescribed for menstrual cramps, acne, mid-cycle spots or other hormone-related aggravations. But it's important to become familiar with your own cycle, if you don't become pregnant straight away, and to see these hormonal fluctuations as positive signs of your fertility.

It used to be thought sensible for women coming off the Pill, or stopping any other form of hormonal contraception, to wait a few months for their cycle to regularize and also to allow time for these artificial hormones to be excreted from the body. However, it is now advised not to wait, especially as there is some evidence to show that coming off the Pill kick-starts a woman's hormonal activity and may actually encourage conception.

The other advantage with being familiar with your own cycle, and what its ups and downs might be, as well as its regularity or otherwise, means that if there are problems with conception you have a baseline for considering what those problems might be.

For some women, once they know what to look for, their personal indicators of fertility are very clear-cut – it's that, 'Oh, yes...' moment. Fertility UK statistics illustrate that over 60 per cent of couples who contact a fertility awareness practitioner via www.fertilityuk.org do so in order to increase their understanding of the menstrual cycle to help plan a pregnancy.

How long can I expect before my periods return following the Pill?
Delays are not uncommon, especially in women over 30. It really helps to understand your cycle. Initially you may experience some irregularities in your cycle, including cycles that are longer than 35 days. Also, you may not ovulate in all cycles. If you are doing a temperature chart you may not get a rise in temperature – this happens, on average, in 10 per cent of cycles. Some women will have no periods (amenorrhea) or a cycle lasting over 90 days.

Am I more likely to have Polycystic Ovary Syndrome (PCOS) after taking the Pill?
It seems that some women who do come off the Pill and then have irregular cycles are diagnosed with Polycystic Ovary Syndrome. The Pill prevents PCOS, as it prevents ovulation and reduces the hormonal activity that causes PCOS, but there is little evidence to suggest that you are more likely to get PCOS after stopping the Pill, if you have not had it before. However, existing PCOS symptoms may have been masked by the Pill – and so become apparent after stopping.

If I am trying to chart my fertility following the Pill, what can I expect?
The first thing to remember is that there are many different types of Pill – some are combined pills containing oestrogen and progestogen (synthetic progesterone), other hormonal preparations (including pills, patches, injections and contraceptive implants) contain progestogen only. The main effect of oestrogen in pill preparations is to prevent ovulation, while the main effect of progestogen is to cause a thick mucus plug at the cervix, stopping sperm from getting through.

After stopping the Pill (or other hormonal contraceptive products) there will be much variability in how long it takes for full ovulation to return and for cervical secretions to return to their most fertile characteristics. Normally these things happen very quickly after stopping contraceptive pills (or sometimes, of course, even if you miss out on taking your pill regularly!), but sometimes it takes several months to a year or more for the return of full fertility.

After stopping the Pill it is possible that you may immediately have regular cycles with clear-cut fertility signs, but many women experience irregular cycles – often longer cycles – and there may be disruptions to the normal pattern of secretions because the progestogen in your pill has kept your cervix tightly closed and plugged with a sticky white mucus to stop sperm from entering. It can take a while for the cervix to start producing the more sperm-friendly wetter, clearer secretions again in good quantities.

If you are recording your temperature, there may be some cycles with no temperature rise (possibly indicating the absence of ovulation), while other cycles may show a rise in temperature but it may occur fewer than 10 days before the next period starts (indicating a short luteal phase). If this is the case, your cycle would not be fertile as there would be insufficient time for implantation to succeed.

Many women report heavier and brighter red bleeding after stopping the Pill – this can be quite alarming. Hormone-withdrawal bleeding which you get during the pill-free interval is much lighter and pinker than the fresh red bleeding of a normal period. If you are concerned, do talk to your doctor.

How will I know if I am ovulating or not?

It is not possible to tell from cervical secretions, temperature or LH kits whether ovulation is happening or not. The build-up to the wetter, clearer secretions indicates that ovulation is approaching, LH kits generally show that ovulation is imminent, and the rise in temperature may be a sign that ovulation has occurred – however none of these signs is conclusive.

Aim to have as much sex as possible at any time you see any cervical secretions – this gives sperm the best possible chance to start their journey!

It will be hard at first to recognize your individual pattern. If you are concerned about a delay in conceiving, of course you should speak to your doctor in the first instance.

For many women there is a wealth of minor signs and symptoms that can help identify their fertile times. Let's take a look at some of these.

Increased Libido

An increase in libido – of course this is also related to other emotional, social and physical factors, but for many women trying to get pregnant, increased sexual interest is an indicator of hormonal changes around the time of ovulation.

Mid-cycle Abdominal Pain

Because the ovarian follicle enlarges, prior to ovulation, by up to 23mm, and ruptures at ovulation, it's not surprising that some women become aware of a sharp twinge or dull ache on either the right- or left-hand side of their lower abdomen, about halfway between the navel and hip bone and halfway between the navel and pubic bone. This can last for anything up to a couple of hours, and may be combined with a crampy feeling, not dissimilar to menstrual cramps, which may be because of the swollen ovary or the extending of the womb and Fallopian tubes, caused by the increase in oestrogen. The actual cause of the pain is still not known – the most likely culprit, as identified by research carried out in Germany, is related to a very slight bleed into the peritoneum as the follicle ruptures.

With other fertility awareness already in place, many women can easily identify this time of peak fertility, which can be an extremely useful indicator. Mid-cycle, or ovulation pain is also referred to as *mittelschmertz* – though it has to be mentioned that research has shown that of all the subjective indicators of fertility, this one is the most varied in relation to ovulation (when studied on ultrasound scans).

Breast Tenderness

This is also an indicator, often unwelcome for many women, that they are about to ovulate. Tenderness leading up to ovulation tends to be tingling in nature, because of the oestrogen effect. Tenderness that comes on towards the end of the cycle, influenced by the progesterone effect, is usually characterized by a heavy and full feeling, rather than tingling.

Spotting

In a very few women it is normal for them to experience a little mid-cycle spotting, or to have pink-coloured cervical mucus because of this spotting. For those women this is an indicator of peak fertility, but because it is so uncommon is not often listed as a fertility indicator. In addition, any mid-cycle spotting or bleeding must be reported to your doctor and checked out, as it can be an indicator of infection or disease. Make sure you are up to date on your smear tests.

What if my LH surge does not relate to my secretions?

An LH kit shows that ovulation is about to happen (within the next 24 hours). Cervical secretions give you about 5 days' warning. To optimize your chances of pregnancy, have sex from the time your secretions start (this is the start of the fertile time). Normally the LH kit will become positive after you have had fertile secretions for a few days. Do not wait for a positive result from a urine sample – by the time you get this you are nearing the end of your fertile time. If you do have a positive LH test, continue to have regular sex for at least two days afterwards.

What if all of the LH tests are negative?

This can be very alarming for women, as you only get five test sticks, and if you have no idea about your fertility you won't even be sure of when to start testing. If a woman has an irregular cycle, ovulation could vary anywhere between days 14 and 28, or even earlier or later than this, making it very hard to pinpoint exactly.

The LH sticks may not work for some women, for example some women over 40 may have higher LH readings. Similarly, some women with PCOS may have raised LH levels. If you use the sticks and find that you do not see any negative days – i.e. all your test results are positive – this may be a sign that you have an abnormally high LH level throughout your cycle. This should be checked by your doctor.

Ovulation does not occur in every cycle. It can be affected by factors such as age, the amount of time since you last gave birth, whether you are breastfeeding, how long it has been since you stopped taking the Pills, your body weight and stress levels. It is quite common not to ovulate in around 1 out of every 10 cycles. If you have two or more consecutive cycles where you do not think you have ovulated, see your doctor.

Why is my doctor going to check my progesterone levels?

Your doctor may do a progesterone test to check for ovulation. This is commonly called a Day 21 progesterone test. Doctors aim to test for the hormone progesterone about halfway through the second half (luteal) phase of your cycle – and for a woman with a cycle of 28 days, halfway between day 14 and 28 is Day 21. However, this only gives an accurate reading if your cycles are 28 days long. For shorter cycles the test may need to be done earlier, for longer ones, later. To time this test more accurately – and if you are aware of your fertile secretions – aim to get the test done about a week after your peak secretion day (i.e. one week after the secretions change back from being clear, wet and stretchy to being thick, white or dry again). If you are taking your temperature regularly, aim to have your progesterone test about six to seven days after your temperature rose to its higher level.

If you are told that a progesterone test shows you are not ovulating, this is not necessarily all doom and gloom. It simply means that you did not ovulate during that particular cycle. The test may need to be repeated to get an idea of whether this was an isolated incidence or a common occurrence for you.

What does it mean if my secretions do not get to the raw egg white stage?
Some women never notice egg-white type secretions yet conceive quite normally. It is the quality of the secretions high up in the cervix that count for the sperm. Avoid feeling inside your cervix to check for secretions, as this can be quite drying. As we get older the amount and quality of secretions reduces – so you may have noticed that these secretions were more abundant in your younger years. A reduction in secretions could be related purely to your observations – or may be related to slightly lower oestrogen levels. Many women never see the really stretchy type of secretion – but feel wetter only.

Can I use saliva, KY jelly or egg whites for lubrication during intercourse if I am dry?
No, unfortunately saliva has been found to be quite detrimental to sperm. In laboratory conditions, sperm cannot swim if they are in contact with saliva or any other lubricant – either water- or oil-based – all of these have some effect on sperm motility (movement). Although this has not been tested in women (and would be quite hard to study!), one has to assume that the effect would be the same in the body. Saliva of

course contains an enzyme, ptyalin, which starts the digestive process – digesting carbohydrates – so this is not good news for the sugars contained in sperm or their swimming fluids!

Lubricating gels block the sperm. Egg whites are protein and can trigger an allergic reaction in some women.

I don't seem to have many secretions, yet they seemed plentiful when I was younger. Is this common?

Yes, as we get older the quantity and quality of our cervical secretions are reduced. This is one of the reasons why fertility rates are lower in older women. The other factor is often that when young we are often unaware of the significance of these secretions and may even be quite alarmed by them. Sometimes women feel the secretions are a sign of infection – or that they may have damaged themselves somehow.

It is also common for women to report that as soon as they start to look out for the secretions, they no longer seem to see them. The amount of secretions will vary from woman to woman and sometimes from one cycle to the next in the same woman. If you are having sex around your fertile time (which is of course pretty vital) then often some of your natural secretions will get mixed in with the seminal fluid, which then comes away a few minutes after you have sex (even if you are lying flat) and can give you the impression that you've fewer secretions than you really have.

What if I spot between periods?

This depends on when the spotting is occurring. The first thing to remember is that ANY unusual bleeding or spotting must be checked out by your doctor. It is important to keep your cervical smears up to date, as these check not only for pre-cancerous changes but also for signs of infection.

If any spotting has been checked out medically and you are told that there is no concern medically, the following information may be help-ful. Some women get spotting towards the end of a period – this may be quite normal as the period dries up. Some women have spotting lead-ing into a period. This should be recorded at the end of the cycle – with the new cycle (Day 1) starting on the first day that you notice fresh red bleeding. If you consistently get some spotting for a day or so before your red bleed starts (pre-menstrual spotting), this may be an indication that your progesterone level is falling and may require medical help.

Very occasionally women who are observing cervical secretions report slight spotting tingeing the wet stretchy secretions – this is noth-ing to be concerned about (provided you are having regular smear tests) and may simply be due to the fact that you are more aware of your secretions than ever before!

Some women notice a tiny spot or so of blood (or even more) around the time implantation is occurring – so this could be a very positive sign.

I seem to have a long cycle and have secretions nearly all of my cycle.
Although most women report that they are dry immediately after a period and when approaching the next period, some will observe secretions for most, if not all, of the cycle. Again, if you suspect any infection, get this checked by your doctor.

Quite a common reason for secretions throughout the cycle is a cervical eversion (where the inner lip of the cervix protrudes onto the outside of the cervix, causing an increase in the wetter type of secre-tions). This is more common after you have been on the Pill, or after pregnancy or miscarriage, and may go away of its own accord. See your doctor or practice nurse, who will be able to see if there are any signs of an eversion. It is not necessary to treat this, unless the secretions are causing trouble with increased wetness. Your doctor will be able to advise you.

Women can learn to distinguish cervical secretions more easily if they get expert help from a health professional trained in fertility awareness methods – such help can be found at www.fertilityuk.org.

When I take my temperature it seems to be very low, and never gets above 35.5°C. Is this a problem?

If your temperature does not seem to fit on the scale of the usual fertility chart, the most likely reason is either a faulty thermometer or inexperience in taking your temperature. It may be worth consulting a trained fertility practitioner. If you have a very low waking temperature – and you are sure you are taking it correctly – then do check this with your doctor. If you also have other symptoms such as tiredness, or are feeling the cold, then there may be a thyroid problem. Your doctor will be able to check your thyroid function as part of other hormone testing.

I suffer from PCOS and have very irregular cycles. How can I know when I should have sex?

This is difficult. Many women with PCOS have erratic ovulation and confusing fertility symptoms, and can have patchy secretions throughout the month due to erratic hormone levels. Ovulation kits will be of no value if your level of LH is raised or high, as it sometimes is when you have this condition.

Plan to have frequent, regular sex throughout the month. I have seen many women conceive with PCOS; the good news is 70 per cent conceive naturally and 20 per cent conceive with the help of appropriate medication.

If you are older, have been diagnosed with PCOS and have made all the necessary lifestyle changes, don't leave it too long before you consult with your doctor about problems getting pregnant – it's possible you may not be ovulating.

understanding male fertility

Male Reproductive System

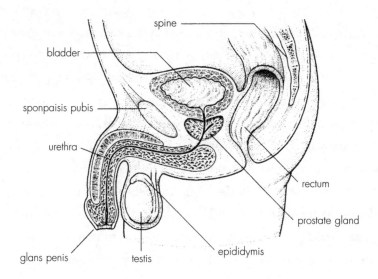

spine

bladder

sponpaisis pubis

urethra

rectum

prostate gland

glans penis

testis

epididymis

A man's general health is just as important to conception as a woman's, although this often gets overlooked by fertility experts, who tend to be gynaecologists and obstetricians – specialists in female, not male, reproductive health. And your health is never more important than when you and your partner are trying to conceive. Very often, problems in conception are thought to be wholly the woman's, but this is not the case. When a couple have a problem with conception, the problem is only with the woman in around 35 to 40 per cent of cases and with the man between 30 and 35 per cent of the time. Problems that arise from combined difficulties in both partners account for the other 25 to 35 per cent of cases.

I do think that, slowly, the message is getting through: The health of the sperm is just as important as a woman's gynaecological health when it comes to conception. At our clinic we will offer a semen analysis straight away; if you focus all clinical attention on the woman, valuable fertility time may be wasted.

Unlike women, men do not have cycles which could alert them to the fact that there may be problems – so very often it can come as a real shock when the results of a semen analysis are poor. And semen analysis is only part of the story: the sperm may look fantastic but there may be infections or DNA fragmentation, which will not show up on semen analysis. Specimens sent to standard general microbiology or pathology labs may not receive immediate attention, and morphology assessment in particular (see page 286) may be inadequate, giving false or misleading results. We have seen this happen so many times.

Twenty-five per cent of male infertility remains unexplained. Sperm counts have been steadily declining over the last 50 years. Scientific evidence clearly points towards our constant exposure to toxins in our everyday modern lives, contributing to our reproductive downfall. These factors are known to affect male reproductive function seriously, and may well contribute to this high number of unexplained cases.

Insufficient emphasis is put on the contribution of lifestyle factors to sperm quality and male infertility. Infertility is multi-factorial and, in many cases, the severity of male infertility is exacerbated by lifestyle factors, which can and should be addressed to optimize whatever fertility potential there is. Even if the semen analysis is good, good sperm genetic health and metabolic fitness can always be improved by cutting down on the lifestyle factors that are known to harm the sperm, and eating a good healthy diet to reduce oxidative damage to the sperm.

Sperm Production

Sperm are produced in the seminiferous tubules of each testis. The two testes are contained in the scrotal sac, next to the penis. Unlike women, who are born with around 2 million immature eggs in their ovaries, although they don't begin to mature and ovulation doesn't occur until after puberty, a man doesn't produce sperm at all until puberty, when his reproductive hormones become active.

Hormones are sometimes called the 'chemical messengers' of the body. Secreted by a gland in one part of the body, hormones are transported via the bloodstream to another area of the body, where they have an effect. At puberty, for both men and women, an area of the brain called the hypothalamus starts secreting gonadotrophin-releasing hormones, which cause the pituitary gland to produce two other hormones: follicle-stimulating hormone (FSH) and luteinizing hormone (LH). When these two hormones are produced, the gonads – testes in men, ovaries in women – are stimulated, to produce sperm in the man and to stimulate ovulation in a woman. The average age for male puberty is between 12 and 14, although this can vary quite widely and is influenced to some degree by genetic make-up, race and diet. Hormonal stimulation of the testes leads to the production of sperm and, as long as the necessary hormones are available and at the correct levels, and there is no disease or illness affecting production, this is a continuous process from puberty onwards.

The other effect of FSH and LH on the testes is to stimulate the production of testosterone, within the testes, responsible for the development of male characteristics like facial, armpit and pubic hair, and body hair in general. The voice also deepens as the testosterone makes the Adam's apple at the front of the neck enlarge. Muscle tissue is increased and strengthened, and mood is also influenced – not least in promoting sexual interest. Some men seem to produce more testosterone than others, but this doesn't mean they are more fertile than other men. Testosterone is responsible for the secondary sex characteristics described above, and isn't particularly an indicator of the quality of sperm or a man's fertility.

The process by which sperm are formed in the testes takes around 100 days – 74 for the sperm to develop, and then another 20-30 days to reach maturity, which is what you have to allow before you can expect to see any improvement in sperm quality or quantity. But as sperm production is happening continuously, a man is continuously fertile, unlike a woman who is only fully fertile for about eight hours during each one of her fertility cycles!

Within the testes, the sperm start their journey through the thousands of tiny, coiled seminiferous tubules. Sperm start as spermatocytes, primary cells that divide and develop into spermatids, which are immature, tail-less sperm. During their journey along the seminiferous tubules, where they are nourished by the sertoli cells that line the tubules, each spermatid grows a head that contains all the chromosomal material. Chromosomes carry all of a man's genetic material ready to pass on to a child, including the chromosome (usually referred to as the sex chromosome) that decides whether a baby will be a boy or a girl. Whereas every one of a woman's eggs contains the genetic material for a girl (the X chromosome), a man's sperm will contain either an X chromosome or a Y chromosome (for a boy).

As well as growing a head during their 74-day development, the sperm form a middle piece that contains the energy source, and a tail. It is the mid-piece of the sperm, with its energy source, which is responsible for the tail's ability to move and transport the sperm independently. Without a properly functioning tail, sperm may swim around in circles rather than forward in a straight line, or may not swim at all.

From the seminiferous tubules, the maturing sperm move into the epididymis, which is a long tube, around 18 feet in length but only a three-hundredth of an inch in diameter, which is coiled and situated at the back of the testicle.

Once produced, sperm then move up into the vas deferens, the tubes that eventually feed into the urethra and on through the penis, via the ejaculatory duct. Here, the sperm mix with secretions from the seminal vesicles and the prostate gland to form the seminal fluid. Once combined, the sperm and seminal fluid are referred to as semen. The secretions of the prostate gland are alkaline, which helps to neutralize the acidity of the woman's vagina, and protect the sperm. The vas deferens travel from the testes out of the scrotum and through the lower abdomen via the groin, then around to a point underneath the bladder where they join the urethra. They hold an astonishing amount of sperm: it would take around 30 ejaculations to empty the vas deferens of their full load!

Only around 20 per cent of semen is sperm. The seminal fluid that combines with sperm to form semen is composed of more than 22 different chemicals, including sugar, vitamins C, E and B$_{12}$, prostaglandins (which help stimulate muscle contractions and the dilatation of blood vessels), the minerals zinc, potassium and sulphur, and essential fatty acids (namely DHA). Altogether, ejaculate consists of around 2 to 4 ml of semen, which is quite viscous at first but then liquefies after about 10 minutes. Sperm need to be nourished by this liquid on their journey, and protected from the acidic environment of the woman's vagina, before any of them can reach an egg. Around 250 million sperm are ejaculated each time, but it takes only one to fertilize an egg.

Why this enormous quantity of sperm? Only a certain proportion – and this varies from man to man – will be normal, active enough and capable of fertilizing an egg in the first place. Then, because the woman's vagina is acidic, and hostile to sperm, treating it as it would any other 'foreign body' and attempting to get rid of it, as it would an infection, this also reduces the available sperm. From here, only around a million sperm will actually get as far as the woman's cervix, and only around 200 of these, at most, will reach the woman's Fallopian tube, to fertilize an egg.

If you then consider how many of the remaining sperm are actually of a good enough quality to fertilize an egg – and in sperm analysis only a maximum of 20 per cent pass this test – it's no wonder that fertilization can be a tricky business. And even if fertilization does occur, if the sperm responsible is faulty in some way then development of the fertilized egg can't continue, and miscarriage may be the outcome.

A Good Diet

When you consider what sperm need to develop, and the journey they have to undertake in order to stand a chance of fertilizing an egg, it's easier to understand why good health in a man is just as important as in a woman when it comes to making babies.

The good news is that, because of the continuous 100-day cycle of sperm production, it is possible to improve sperm's quality relatively easily, by making the necessary health and lifestyle changes.

While the Nutrition chapter (see page 89) offers general guidelines, it is worth mentioning here, too, that when it comes to the sort of adequate nutrition that makes a difference, there is no point grabbing a general multi-vitamin, or an expensive supplement, unless you know what you're getting and what you need. Before that, it's worth looking at your general diet and how to improve it.

Generally speaking, the fresher and less processed the food you eat, the better. Many people advocate organic foods, and there is a good argument for this. In one Danish study, an unexpectedly high sperm count was found among organic farmers. Their sperm count was twice as high as that of a control group of blue-collar workers. But it's tricky, because if it's a choice between organic beans flown in from Kenya that have taken five days to get to your supermarket shelf and have then sat in your fridge for two days, and some locally-produced beans that are not organic but were picked yesterday, you might want to choose the latter, as the vitamin and mineral content of the fresher food will be higher, and washing it carefully will help remove chemical and pesticide residues.

Now is not the time to go on some extreme weight-loss diet, either. Some men opt for high-protein diets to lose weight, but we have noticed anecdotally that men following this type of diet have poor sperm. There's evidence to show that extreme diets, like the low-carb ones in such favour these days, increase the body's acidity if not actually leaving you malnourished, which won't be good for sperm production. Better to adjust the balance of what you eat, increase your exercise a little, and reduce your weight that way.

Ideally, you should follow the guidelines set out in the Nutrition and Lifestyle chapters.

Try also to eat a proportion of your foods, especially fresh fruit and vegetables, raw. And when you do cook, try steaming and grilling rather than boiling or frying, which will preserve more of your food's nutritional value.

It is probably a good idea to cut out all highly processed foods, if you can, as they are alarmingly high in hidden fats, sugars and chemical preservatives. In addition, the nutritional content of food is greatly reduced during processing. Opt for whole foods where you can.

If this feels rather overwhelming, start gradually, introducing a different change into your diet week by week as you adjust.

Water
When it comes to what you drink (and alcohol is covered separately: see page 62), make sure you are not over-doing your caffeine intake.

Caffeine is mildly addictive, so if you are used to drinking a lot it may take a while to kick the habit. There is also some evidence to show that if a man has a high caffeine intake before conception, the risk of premature birth is increased. Tea contains tannin, which is less of a stimulant than caffeine, but excess quantities will deplete you of iron.

Most men do not drink enough water. Sperm need to swim!

Start changing your drinking habits first of all by increasing your water intake – most of us drink too little, generally, to be adequately hydrated.

What Do Sperm Need?

There is a lot of research available now about free radical damage to sperm, but thankfully there's a lot you can do to improve this. To produce sperm your body needs a good intake of certain nutrients, which may need supplementing if they are not readily available from your diet. Research has shown that certain vitamins and minerals improve overall sperm counts – I've seen it many times. It is important, however, to remember **not to exceed the recommended daily allowance (RDA) of any one item,** even if you have heard that it might be beneficial, unless under supervision from a health professional. An excess of one item can deplete others, so a balance is needed.

Also see the Nutrition chapter for more advice on how to improve your diet to increase the chances of conception.

Vitamin C

A well-known antioxidant, under normal conditions vitamin C protects sperm from oxidative damage, and certainly improves sperm quality in men who smoke. However, some men have a condition of their sperm called 'agglutination' where sperm clump together and fertility is reduced. In these cases, vitamin C supplementation of up to 1 gram a day helps reduce agglutination – and was shown to increase fertility in one group of men in a controlled study.

Zinc

Semen is rich in zinc, and men lose a certain amount of this mineral per ejaculate. Zinc is often referred to as the 'fertility mineral' and its presence in foods like oysters, which are said to have aphrodisiac properties, may reinforce this idea! Certainly an insufficiency of zinc can lead to both reduced numbers of sperm and impotence in some men. It has also been found that the levels of zinc in the semen of infertile men are of a lower level than in fertile men. Numerous studies have been done, and some of the results seem to conflict, but overall there is enough evidence to suggest that for men with poor sperm quality, sperm count and sperm motility, a supplement of zinc can help.

In areas of the country where the copper content of water is naturally high there may be a general zinc deficiency, as these two minerals have to be in balance: an excess of copper can reduce zinc. Conversely, where long-term zinc supplementation is recommended, then supplementation with copper is needed.

Vitamin B$_{12}$

Necessary to maintain fertility, there are studies that have shown an improvement in sperm motility where oral vitamin B$_{12}$ was given. In the latter case, around 60 per cent of those men who received an oral supplement of vitamin B$_{12}$ (1,500 mcg per day of methylcobalamin) had improved sperm counts.

Vitamin E

Certainly a deficiency in vitamin E, in animals, leads to infertility. In one human trial, the giving of 100-200 iu of vitamin E daily to both partners led to a significant increase in fertility. Vitamin E seems to reduce the amount of free-radical damage done to cells. Supplementing reduces the amount of oxidative stress on sperm cells, although it should be said that the research is at a preliminary stage and needs further work before a definite case for sperm improvement can be made.

Co-enzyme Q10

This is a nutrient used by the body's cells in the production of energy. Its exact role in the production of sperm isn't known, but there is evidence to show that as little as 10mg a day over a two-week period will improve both sperm count and motility. In one study, where men with low sperm counts were given 60mg a day over a three-month period, although no significant change was observed in most measures of sperm quality and quantity, in-vitro fertilization rates improved significantly.

Selenium

This is an essential trace mineral that acts with the antioxidant vitamins A, C and E, and is found in large quantities in Brazil nuts. In one double-blind study of infertile men, supplementation of 100 mcg per day of selenium for three months significantly increased sperm motility, but not sperm count.

Calcium

The motility of sperm is partly determined by the concentration of calcium in semen, and this mineral is also a key regulator of human sperm function. However, although we know it is important there has been no evidence to confirm that a calcium deficiency causes male infertility. Neither is there any evidence to show that calcium supplementation improves male infertility.

Pycnogenol

Pycnogenol (French maritime pine bark extract) is a natural antioxidant that has been found useful in maintaining the health of blood vessel walls and circulation. It works, at least in part, by subduing free radicals. A preliminary study recently presented at the 54th Annual Meeting of the American Society for Reproductive Medicine/16th World Congress on Fertility and Sterility in San Francisco reported the findings of Dr Scott J. Roseff and his colleagues at the West Essex Center for Advanced Reproductive Endocrinology in West Orange, New Jersey. In the study, four 'subfertile' male patients took daily supplements of Pycnogenol® for three months. These men had had relatively high numbers of deformed sperm, as well as low sperm counts and activity. After 90 days, the percentage of structurally normal sperm – that is, non-deformed sperm – increased by an average of 99 per cent. 'The number of deformed sperm went down and the number of normal sperm went up,' Dr Roseff said. 'The increase in morphologically (structurally) normal sperm is significant, although this is just a preliminary study. Pycnogenol could enable some couples to forego expensive in-vitro fertilization in favour of simpler and less expensive intrauterine insemination.'

SAMe (S-adenosyl-L-methionine)

SAMe is manufactured in the body from the amino acid methionine, with the aid of the co-factors vitamin B_{12} and folic acid, and is essential in the production of the nucleic acids DNA and RNA and other proteins. Although its use as a supplement has been mainly for those suffering depression, migraines, osteoarthritis and liver disease, some preliminary research has shown that SAMe may also increase sperm activity in infertile men, although it's too early for this to be conclusive. Also, as this amount is over the RDA, please consult a qualified nutritionist before you take it.

Arginine

Another amino acid, arginine is found in many foods needed to enhance sperm production. Research, of which most is still in its preliminary stages, has shown that supplementation with L-arginine over several months increased sperm count, quality and fertility. As a supplement it is also an immune-system enhancer and powerful growth-hormone stimulant, while also playing a role in circulation and sexual function. In some susceptible individuals it can also reactivate a latent herpes infection, and shouldn't be used by people with diabetes.

L-carnitine

Another amino acid-like substance, made by the body and also found in meat, L-carnitine is responsible for utilizing fat in the energy centres of the body's cells, and is essential for the formation of lean muscle in the body. It also appears to be necessary for the normal functioning of sperm cells. In preliminary studies, giving an L-carnitine supplement for four months helped to normalize sperm motility in men with poor sperm quality. In another trial, acetylcarnitine was used, and a supplement of 4 grams a day proved useful for male infertility caused by immobile sperm. However, again, this amount is well over the RDA, and should not be taken without supervision.

DHA

So important for sperm. The semen contains high levels of DHA. Animals fed a diet lacking in DHA showed decreased levels in their sperm.

For more about eating well to increase fertility, see the Nutrition chapter.

Other Important Nutrients

These include folic acid – a nutrient just as important for men as it is for women – saw palmetto and NAC. As always, please do consult a qualified nutritionist for more information about dosages and how all these nutrients can assist fertility.

VITAMIN E	SELENIUM	VITAMIN C	ZINC	ARGININE	CARNITINE	VITAMIN B$_{12}$	FOLIC ACID
Nut & seed oils Nuts & seeds Wheat-germ & Wheat-germ oil Whole grains Eggs Green leafy vegetables	Brazil nuts Wheat-germ Oats Garlic & onions Barley Butter Smoked herring Brown rice Whole grains	Citrus fruits Kiwi fruit Straw-berries Black-currants Red pepper Broccoli Cabbage Brussels sprouts Melon Mango Water-cress	Meat Fish Chicken Eggs Pumpkin/Sunflower seeds Whole grains Beans & pulses Ginger root	Nuts esp. Walnuts Almonds Brazil nuts Beans Lentils	Beef Pork Lamb Dairy products	Meat Fish esp. trout, salmon, sardines Eggs Cheese esp. Edam	Green leafy vegetables Beans Lentils Asparagus Oatmeal Dried figs Avocado

Environment and Lifestyle Factors Affecting Sperm Production

I think the way we live and our environment have definitely had an effect on the decline of sperm. Laptop computers, solvents, chemicals – such as those you may use for a hobby or as part of your work – 'gender-bending' environmental oestrogens, paints, pesticides, plastics, aluminium – all of these affect fertility. So, too, can natural substances such as genistein, a compound found in soya products and pulses, and various contaminants in drinking water. In addition, there are factors brought about by the trend towards increasingly sedentary occupations and lack of physical activity, which increase scrotal temperature and affect sperm production, count and motility. All in all, the risks are far greater than they were even 20 years ago.

Much research has been done on animals into the factors that affect reproduction. Until recently, scientists paid little attention to the effects of environmental agents on human reproduction. Chemicals can affect the testes, diminishing or damaging the numbers of sperm, and those found in rubber, solvents and lead have been shown in studies to increase the risk of spontaneous abortion.

We'll now take a brief look at some of the parts of your life that can have an effect on sperm production – more about each of these in the Lifestyle chapter.

Exercise

While regular exercise is a good thing, like anything else if taken to extreme it can be detrimental. In the case of fertility, too much exercise can cause hormone imbalances and increased heat production. Heavy-duty workouts at the gym, marathon training or long-distance cycling make too much of a demand on the body's energy, distracting it from sperm production. If you are using up lots of vitamins, minerals and calories in supporting your muscles and major organs such as the lungs, heart and brain, then there's going to be less available for the production of sperm!

There has also been some research done on the effects of cycling, where there are extended periods of sitting on a hard, narrow bicycle seat. Numbness and pressure on the testicles, prostate and urethra have resulted in prostate problems, impotence or tumours. The incidence of impotence has been found to be four times higher in cyclists than non-cyclists, probably as a result of the continued pressure reducing blood flow.

Cross-country cycling is potentially the most hazardous, according to a German study that made an ultrasound comparison between the testicles of 45 mountain bikers, who cycled for at least two hours a day for six days a week, and 31 non-cycling medical students. Forty-three of the cyclists, compared to five of the non-cyclists, had scrotal abnormalities. Researchers also found that hard saddles can reduce a man's libido by up to 80 per cent, because of the reduction of the blood flow to the scrotal area. Although these are extreme examples, the recommendation is that hard bike saddles should be avoided, padded cycling shorts should be worn, the saddle should be correctly adjusted – either horizontal or pointing downwards at the front – and men should make sure to get off the saddle regularly.

When it comes to regular exercise, choose something that also incorporates some element of stress-reduction and relaxation. If you want to work out in a gym, balance it with swimming, or if you play competitive sport regularly, try something more relaxing such as walking or t'ai chi. Most of us live quite sedentary lives, not using our bodies as they were designed; the knock-on effect can be an accumulation of physical and mental stress, in addition to excess weight.

Stress

A certain amount of stress is inevitable in life. It keeps us on our toes, and many challenges in our work and home life can have an element of pleasurable stress, when a nice event is anticipated, a new skill is mastered or a deadline completed. Stress, however, can build up in an insidious way until it starts to affect our physical well-being, especially if it is constant. Although we apparently adjust to raised levels of stress, it is only because our bodies compensate, but at a cost to our physical health. As preparation for parenthood – one of life's most stressful activities – learning how to reduce the stress in your life now could pay dividends later! (See Lifestyle chapter for help with this.)

Alcohol, Tobacco and Drugs

Often, one of the ways in which we compensate for a busy, stressful and demanding life is to relax with the aid of recreational drugs. Having outlined what sperm need for healthy production, and how they are consistently being produced, it's easy to see how what you eat, drink, smoke or otherwise ingest may have an impact on the production and quality of sperm.

Alcohol

The odd glass of wine or pint of beer (later diluted with lots of water) is not a problem. It is binge drinking that is the issue. Alcohol is a poison and slows down cell division. Two months later a binge will still be affecting the sperm.

There is no reason to suppose that drinking up to the recommended allowance for men (21 units a week) will have a negative effect – as long as everything else is in balance and you and your partner are having no problems conceiving. A unit of alcohol is one pub-sized measure of spirits, glass of wine, or half-pint of ordinary-strength beer, lager or cider. Whatever you think you drink over the course of a week, it's worth keeping a record over a couple of weeks – you may be surprised how it mounts up, especially if you're in the habit of using alcohol as a means of relaxing after a stressful day. Also, it's worth remembering that 21 units a week may not be OK for all men – everyone is different and has a different tolerance.

If you have any reason to think that drinking alcohol might be contributing to difficulties in conceiving, you should really consider not drinking at all. This is particularly important if your general health is consistently below par, your diet is lacking in adequate nutrients, or you know your sperm production is poor.

Heavy drinking is definitely bad for both your health and your sperm. An excessive intake of alcohol has been shown to depress sperm production. In addition, the other obvious effect of high alcohol intake on fertility – impotency or 'brewer's droop' – will certainly make conception tricky!

One of the by-products of alcohol breakdown is acetaldehyde, which has a toxic effect on sperm. It can cause chromosomal abnormalities during the time at which sperm are forming, so bear in mind the 100-day cycle of sperm production. The formation of the tails of each sperm can be adversely affected by alcohol, so their ability to move properly will be diminished. Regular, excessive drinking will also restrict the liver's detoxing ability, making a build-up of toxins more likely.

People who drink heavily tend also to have a poor nutritional status, as not only can alcohol deplete the B vitamins, for example, but those who drink to excess tend not to eat regularly or well. As alcoholic drinks are highly calorific, there is a tendency towards weight gain, too. Binge-drinking at the weekend is easy to slip into if you feel under stress, but in the long term will do little to ease the stress of trying to conceive.

Take control of your drinking, with professional help if necessary – around 80 per cent of male alcoholics are sterile – but otherwise by cutting down or moderating your intake. Have only a couple of pints on alternate nights during the week, no spirits, and wine only with meals, for example. Spend the time you previously spent drinking socially at some sort of recreational activity that helps you relax. The great news is that most of the effects of alcohol on sperm production are reversible! So start now, and be ready to go in a hundred days' time.

Tobacco
While we all know that smoking is an unhealthy pastime, understanding how detrimental its effects are, especially on fertility, may finally help you see the point of giving up.

Smoking doubles the amount of free-radical damage in the body, robbing it of the important antioxidants vitamin C and selenium, while also reducing levels of zinc. Smoking increases the intake of lead, and cadmium, both highly toxic to body cells.

Smoking also reduces your oxygen intake, making cell replication – on which sperm production has to rely – less efficient. At the same time, numerous other chemicals – up to 30 that can adversely affect fertility – are being inhaled. Men who smoke are likely to have:

- decreased sperm density
- decreased sperm count
- less motile sperm
- an increase in abnormal sperm
- reduced testosterone
- children with increased risk of developing cancer.

This list is enough to make anyone give up!

Tobacco is highly addictive, so giving up can be tricky for many people, however well motivated. Seek help and support if necessary, and remember – the first week is the worst, so find a time to give up when you are more relaxed and away from your usual smoking triggers, if possible. Smoking is also an appetite depressant, so many people worry that if they give up they will put on weight, but if you take a careful look at balancing your diet and including a little extra regular exercise, you should be able to avoid this.

Cannabis

While smoking marijuana is seen as being relatively innocuous, when it comes to sperm production persistent cannabis smoking is very bad news. The active ingredient of cannabis, tetrahydrocannabinol, is chemically related to testosterone. Even taken in moderate amounts it accumulates in the testes, where it can cause poor sperm motility, an increase in the number of abnormal sperm and a low sperm count. It also lowers libido.

Cocaine, Opiates, Steroids

If you use cocaine, however infrequently, and want to conceive a baby, you will have to stop. It binds to the sperm, making them less motile, and also causes problems at fertilization. There is also a correlation between cocaine use and birth defects.

Opiates (heroin, morphine) and anabolic steroids affect hormone production.

Prescription Drugs

If you have a long-standing health problem, however minor, or an acute problem that requires prescription medication, you must tell your doctor that you and your partner are trying for a baby. There are a number of drugs that will affect sperm production, and these include steroids and the drugs used to treat ulcers or gout. Some drugs can affect the absorption of certain nutrients from foods.

A number of antibiotics can affect sperm production or motility, so if you are prescribed a course, check with your doctor that these won't have a negative affect on your sperm production. There may be an alternative.

Beta-blockers, commonly used to help control high blood pressure, can cause problems not only with impotence but also by decreasing sperm counts and motility. Some anti-depressants can cause erection difficulties, too.

Medications that Affect Sperm

Generic Name	Used to Treat	Affect on Fertility
Amiodarone	Abnormal heart rhythm	Inflammation of the testicles and epididymis
Chemotherapy	Cancer	Reduces sperm count, quality and motility
Cimetidine	Indigestion, peptic ulcer, acid reflux disease	Affects hormone production and reduces sperm count
Colchicine	Gout	May severely reduce sperm count
Digoxin	Heart failure, abnormal heart rhythm	Affects hormone production
Erythromycin	Chest infections	May reduce sperm count
Gentamicin	Bacterial infections	Reduces sperm count
Hormonal therapies	Various	May disrupt other hormone production
Ketoconazole	Fungal infections	Reduces sperm count
Methotrexate	Some cancers, arthritis	Reduces sperm count
Nitrofurantoin	Urinary tract infection	Reduces sperm count
Phenytoin	Epilepsy	Reduces sperm quality and motility
Spironolactone	Fluid retention	Affects hormone production
Sulphasalazine	Ulcerative colitis	Reduces sperm count and quality
Tetracycline		Reduces sperm motility
Viagra		Reduces sperm's ability to break through the wall of the egg.

Non-prescription Drugs and Herbal Remedies

Generally speaking, paracetamol is a safe analgesic for headaches, colds and minor pain.

When it comes to herbal remedies, bear in mind that a recent study showed that St John's Wort, echinacea and ginkgo biloba may affect the quality of your sperm and in particular their ability to penetrate an egg. It's worth considering that even the most innocuous and natural-sounding remedy can be quite potent in ways you might not expect.

Physical problems affecting sperm production

Having covered sperm production, and looked a little at how sperm can be affected by what you eat and drink, it's worth also considering how physical problems can have an effect, too. If you think about the vulnerability of the male sex organs, and the distance that has to be travelled for the sperm to reach a woman's egg, you can see that there are opportunities for problems which may be caused by physical damage to the reproductive system.

Injury

A serious blow to the testes can damage them, or the blood flow to them. Occasionally one of the testes can twist on its own spermatic cord, within the scrotal sac. This is called a torsion. The degree of pain felt can vary, but is usually followed by the testis becoming hard and swollen. If a diagnosis isn't made and the torsion isn't rectified within about six hours, permanent damage can result that can leave a man infertile.

Illness

Mumps in children is seldom a problem illness, but in older boys and men the mumps virus can cause 'orchitis' or inflammation of the testes, and lead to infertility. This can also be caused by other infections, including gonorrhoea, and can be excruciatingly painful. The problem is that the infection and consequent inflammation can damage the testes. Even a high fever, above 38.5°C, which can easily occur with flu, can damage sperm production for up to six months.

Overheating

When a baby boy is developing in the womb, the testes develop inside his body. However, for the continued development and correct functioning of the testes they need a cooler temperature and, either before the birth or shortly afterwards, they descend from the abdominal cavity via the groin and into the scrotal sacs.

Sperm production requires an optimum temperature of 32°C, while the body's core temperature is around 37°C. If things get too warm in the groin, this can inhibit sperm production. While there is no need for extreme measures such as ice-packs or cold showers to improve things, there are other steps men can take:

- Avoid wearing very tight pants or trousers. Fortunately, unlike the fashion in the 1970s, looser clothing is now the norm, but underpants tend to be close fitting, so opt for boxer shorts instead. Choose cotton rather than synthetic fibres, too, for added coolness.
- Avoid spending a long time in hot baths, saunas or Jacuzzis. Take a shower where possible instead.
- Long-distance driving can also mean rising temperatures in the groin area. Bear this in mind on long journeys, and take regular breaks. Also, heated seats in cars and lorries are not the best idea if you and your partner are trying to conceive.

Age

There is a change in the quality and production of sperm as men age. The Leydig cells, which produce testosterone, decrease in number over time. The result is a decrease in sperm count and motility, and an increase in the numbers of abnormal sperm. There is also an increase in chromosomal abnormalities in the sperm of older men, which, if they result in conception, can lead to birth defects.

A recent study showed that men aged 35 or older are 50 per cent less likely, over a 12-month period, to achieve conception with a fertile partner than men under 35. This decline in fertility is thought to be attributable to the 'male menopause', when levels of male hormones decrease.

Frequent Sex

A quick word on the myth that frequent sex can deplete or weaken sperm supplies: it's not true! Research has shown that if you and your partner are trying to conceive, the more regular the sex, the more likely you are to achieve this. In Chinese medicine it is believed that the sperm equate to our essence, and that too much sex will weaken it. Don't you believe it!

Many of our clients think that if they abstain or 'save up' the sperm they will be more potent around ovulation. This is not the case. Dr Sheryl Homa likens it to a train arriving at a station: more and more people crowd on, eventually everybody feels ill, there's not enough air and people will start to pass out. The same is true for sperm that are not regularly ejaculated. The numbers may increase to a point, but the quality will deteriorate considerably.

A woman with regular cycles came to the clinic. She had been trying to conceive for three years. Her husband worked abroad for two weeks at a time, only returning home for a few days around the time of his wife's ovulation. Semen analysis on his sperm after 14 days' abstention showed fewer than 5 per cent motile sperm. No wonder they had not been successful!

Assessing a Man's Fertility

It is the case that men discuss their health much less than women do, and are much less aware generally of health issues. When it comes to everyday sexual health, this is perhaps unsurprising: There is no male equivalent to women's monthly cycle to reveal their bodies' inner processes or to affect mental, emotional or physical performance. Men feel pretty much the same all the time unless they are ill or injured. Except for self-evident issues such as impotence, there is no obvious reference point for a man to access his own fertility, or reduced fertility. As Simon Dr Rattenbury, Microbiologist at the Royal Free NHS Trust, says:

> It is a sad but true fact that men don't talk to each other. We tend to bury our collective heads in the sand when it comes to health. I see men from all over the world with various ailments, and I am quite often asked, 'Do other men feel like this?' Women, on the other hand, are far better informed about their health, where to go and what to do if something is wrong. They talk to each other!
>
> Male infertility, or reduced fertility (RD), the term I prefer to use, is no less subject to male indifference: we men leave most of the investigations to our loved ones, with the odd semen analysis to show solidarity with our partners. The male reproductive tract and the substances it produces are complex and subject to many factors that affect our health and ability to conceive. The basics of our health are very important, therefore; a general medical check-up is a prerequisite, and should include a semen analysis.
>
> RF is thought to be a multifactorial disease process with a number of potential contributing factors. The majority of

male infertility cases are due to deficient or reduced sperm production of unknown origin, therefore infections and hormonal, environmental, nutritional and stress factors should all be evaluated. It is important to remember that a semen analysis only gives the basic data and, certainly, results should be treated with caution in the absence of other supporting evidence.

It is therefore important for men to have a full fertility infection screen to include a full semen analysis and a prostate profile.

Semen analysis provides such a valuable insight into the male contribution to conception, and at specific problems, because it can immediately identify those steps that can be taken to improve the quality and quantity of sperm production. In addition, if there is a specific problem that indicates a physical or genetic problem, then further tests can be decided upon.

A man's normal fertility can fluctuate, and is always a matter of degree. So if there is a degree of sub-fertility, where the sperm count is borderline, for example, the reassuring news is that it can usually be improved (see Fertility Work-up chapter).

Our Programme

Our programme for men consists of consultation featuring advice on nutrition and lifestyle, and including:

- Acupuncture
- Hypnosis

The Male Fertility Programme we run at the clinic is lead by Dr Sheryl Homa. Here she explains things in her own words:

When it comes to infertility amongst couples, it is always the women that take the initiative. They are the ones to arrange the doctor's appointments, and the doctors naturally focus on them. Women are usually thoroughly investigated, with blood tests, ultrasound scans and even surgical investigation, and are always referred on to a gynaecologist or fertility clinic if there is a problem. Assessment of the man, on the other hand, usually starts and ends with a semen analysis. If the results are normal, a man is given to understand that there is nothing wrong with him and the problem must lie with the woman. If the results are poor, in a large number of cases the couple are sent to a fertility clinic without further investigation, and some form of assisted conception is offered.

The problem with the general fertility management of the man is that it does not take into account the fact that a semen analysis tells us very little about the ability of the sperm to actually bind to and fertilize the egg, and tells us absolutely nothing about the genetic health of the sperm and whether they can trigger normal healthy embryo development. Indeed, some men may have perfectly lovely-looking sperm under the microscope, but they may have poor genetic integrity.

There may be many reasons for a man's infertility that are best diagnosed by a doctor who specializes in the male genito-urinary tract, namely an andrologist/urologist. Assisted conception treatment for infertility merely circumvents the problem for men; it does not get to the root of their problem to treat it.

It is true to say that a lot of the causes of male infertility cannot be successfully treated; for those that can, it makes much more sense to do this than run head-long into fertility treatment that may not be successful anyway without addressing certain underlying conditions.

Our programme looks at the broader picture, taking into account a variety of factors in addition to the semen analysis. We include state-of-the-art tests to examine sperm genetic health, and recommend that patients have thorough infection screening. We always recommend a follow-up discussion to talk through all of your results in conjunction with the information you provide us regarding your lifestyle, and rec-ommend a plan individually tailored to your needs over a four-month period to maximize your sperm quality and fertil-ity potential. We will always refer you to a urologist if there is anything abnormal. These can be very trying times for you, and we are here to focus on your issues, to listen to you and provide as many answers to your questions as we can.

For more about men's fertility problems and an in-depth look at ways you can help yourself, please take a look at the chapter called Fertility Work-up.

conception

Many couples embarking on getting pregnant today are already in the mindset where they foresee having problems or potential problems. In one sense I see this as a positive change in general attitudes, because it means that more and more couples understand the importance of pre-conceptual care. If they can satisfy themselves that they are doing the right things, most couples then feel happy to go off and try naturally instead of panicking and running down the IVF route. This chapter takes a look at both the myths and the facts around conception.

Myths

You could be forgiven for thinking that getting pregnant is simple: sperm plus egg equals baby. Certainly that is the message you were likely to have been given during any sex education lessons at school – probably with the emphasis on how to avoid getting pregnant. Yet even with this limited understanding it becomes obvious that getting pregnant when you want to is sometimes not that easy.

One thing that will be obvious from reading the chapter on Female Fertility is that a number of things have to come together for the egg to be released, the womb to be receptive, and for conception to occur. Having sex at the appropriate time, or often enough to ensure there are enough live and healthy sperm when ovulation does occur, is only part of the picture. Understanding your own, individual fertility cycle and how getting pregnant is possible are very important.

One of the most common myths is that you shouldn't have sex too often when trying for a baby, as it 'weakens' the sperm. The truth is that the majority of couples seen at our clinic are definitely not having enough sex – and when they are it is seldom at the right time to benefit from a woman's 'fertility window', which lasts from about six days before to one day after ovulation. In general, among couples who are having regular sex – and that means at least two or three times a week – 93 out of 100 will achieve a pregnancy in the first year of trying. This is based on couples having around a 1-in-5 chance of achieving pregnancy each month. So, with 100 fertile couples, 20 will get pregnant the first month, 16 (20 per cent of the remaining 80) in the second month, and so on. But if sex is only occurring weekly, or less, then the chances of conception become very low, if not negligible. This is why one of the first questions I ask a couple is how often they are having sex, whereas I know that in some busy fertility clinics they may not be asked this important question at all! The lack of regular sex (once every Sunday morning ain't gonna get you pregnant!) has even been found to be the 'cause' of unexplained infertility for some couples, and addressing this simple point has been found to eliminate the need for IVF! One thing I always ask couples to look at is their overall pattern of work – shift-work can make things difficult as partners are away from each other at crucial fertile times.

Another myth is that a woman has to have an orgasm to conceive. Although nice, this isn't imperative – far better to relax and enjoy all aspects of lovemaking. There is, however, some evidence to suggest that if ovulation is imminent, the uterine contractions of an orgasm can encourage ovulation to happen. But if ovulation is due in any case, and because sperm live for an average of three days (and sometimes five, or in rare cases even up to seven days), don't panic – make love again and conception may happen after all. And while it is true that the internal contractions of the female orgasm have the effect of helping to draw semen up into the womb and Fallopian tubes, try not to get too hung up about this. You are not frigid if you don't have an orgasm every time you make love, and this isn't a bar to fertility, unless it makes penetration impossible.

Although having fun with different positions during sex keeps the enjoyment alive, there is no real evidence to support the idea that the 'missionary position' gives you a better chance of conceiving. Deep penetration is important – but a lot of women I see start off on top (a position many women find more pleasurable) – I often suggest that this is great – and then change position part-way through so that they end up underneath. Alternatively, a woman and her partner may swap positions together after orgasm, so that she is lying flat and retains fluid! Again, it's important to keep the joy alive in your sex; many women seem to get less pleasure from the missionary position, and their lack of arousal as a result can make penetration more difficult.

If a woman is on her back after her partner's orgasm, the sperm remains in contact with the cervix in the vagina more easily. By the way, there is no need for extreme measures like putting your legs up in the air or doing handstands, but lying still for the next 20 to 30 minutes – without getting up to use the bathroom – will allow time for the sperm to work its way into the womb and Fallopian tubes. Hormones released during sex and orgasm tend to make you feel sleepy and content, so exploit this to help fertilization along.

Most women experience a degree of 'flow-back' of seminal fluid around 30 minutes after ejaculation, when about half the sperm are lost. This concerns many couples because they don't realize that it is normal, but don't fret – even with this loss there are still more than enough sperm left to get the job done!

Maintaining Sexual Pleasure and Intimacy

What can often happen if a couple are beginning to feel rather desperate about getting pregnant is that the joy and romance of their lovemaking go out the window. While there are some aspects of sex that can be pretty basic, without a loving spark it can be difficult for it to be anything more than purely mechanical. It can be extremely hurtful for a woman to feel that she is only of sexual interest to her partner as the potential mother of his children, or for a man to feel he's only being used as stud.

It is very common for me to hear from couples at my clinic that sex has become mechanical; that the woman is only interested in sex when she is ovulating – which causes resentment in her partner – or that they've started rowing about it and fail to have sex at all. In addition, I have seen cases of 'performance anxiety' on the part of the male partner. All the pressure on him to impregnate his partner can lead to impotence. Suddenly, for these couples, sex has become about procreation rather than pleasure, so arousal is difficult, and many couples just can't face it.

Also – and I know it's hard – try above all to keep your perspective about this, and also to make the effort to include lots of non-sexual but intimate time together, to keep the basis of your relationship alive, from which a loving sexuality can emerge. Focus on what it was that first attracted you to each other, and what it was that made you feel that having a baby together would be a lovely idea. Remember what you used to enjoy doing together, as a couple, before life became more mundane – whether that was going for long walks, reading the papers or listening to music together. Take a weekend away, or a holiday – this often works wonders for couples whose desire for having a child has, inadvertently, started to cause feelings of estrangement. Avoid trying desperately to plan that the time away will coincide with what you hope will be your fertile time – this can put extra pressure on you both. This time away is about the two of you, as a couple – not about making babies!

Many things can prevent a couple from having sex. In our time-pressured society, more and more couples are discovering that just finding the time to have sex becomes an additional pressure. Scheduling it into an already busy life, somewhere between work deadlines and entertaining the in-laws, can reduce the intimacy between a couple that makes sex a pleasurable and rewarding part of their relationship.

Sex can also become representative of difficulties between couples. If one partner wants a baby while the other remains ambivalent, this can alter the desire for sex. It can become difficult for a couple to relate to each other, especially sexually.

Here communication is key, and if it has become difficult to talk about these things then it can sometimes be useful to find a third party, a fertility counsellor perhaps, who can help re-open the lines of communication. It's all too easy, when emotions become intense and the desire to achieve a pregnancy is very strong, for couples to have difficulty expressing how they feel to each other.

Modern lifestyles are extremely demanding. Having a baby involves a major life change. For many couples, getting pregnant can become an end in itself, especially if it is proving difficult to accomplish. Some couples, either deliberately or subconsciously, create lifestyles that are very busy and urgent, so there's little time left for the real intimacy and the, frankly, often humdrum nature of relationships. Yet this is exactly what a relationship with a new baby is like: While it can be exciting and magical, it has a lot of extremely dull moments, and also demands a real, day-to-day, up-to-your-elbows-in-nappies intimacy. While you may be able to say 'No' to an increased workload or to demands from family or friends, when a baby needs to be fed there is no way around it. This is why one thing I ask couples is to imagine, as vividly as they possibly can, what having a baby would truly mean to their lives in terms of the time and adjustments that would need to be made. This is important, because an acceptance and accommodation of what it really means to have a baby, even while holding on to the romantic part of the dream, can help it become a reality.

What Needs to Happen?

Yes, the sperm needs to meet the egg, but the first thing to remember is that, although sperm can live for between three and seven days, an egg is only 'fertilizable' for 12 to 24 hours. So timing is important, and this is where fertility awareness comes in. Many women feel embarrassed about not knowing everything on the subject, but they are told so many things by well-meaning friends and relatives that are often irrelevant. A one-off session with a close look at their own cycle is all that some couples need. And in the case of women who have been on the Pill, and therefore have no idea what their cycle is like or what a 'normal' period is for them, this is essential.

A lot of women are advised to wait a few months after they stop taking the Pill before they start trying for a baby. I, however, suggest that women try straight away, as there is some research to suggest that it is easiest to conceive immediately after stopping the Pill, and can get harder as time goes by. This is sometimes referred to as 'rebound fertility'. In one study it was discovered quite by chance that pregnancy occurred twice as often in women having IVF treatment if they had been on the combined oral contraceptive pill beforehand. Prior to embarking on IVF treatment, and depending on a woman's medical history, some doctors prescribe the Pill for a while beforehand to try and increase her potential fertility.

It is also worth taking a nutritional supplement, even before you come off the Pill. Make sure it includes folic acid (the recommendation for a woman contemplating pregnancy is 400 mcg a day to avoid the risk of spinal defects in the foetus). Women with epilepsy and some other medical conditions may need more than 400 mcg daily, so do check with your doctor.

What you also need is for good, healthy sperm to meet the egg, and for the egg itself to be in good condition for fertilization to take place. And for conception of the fertilized egg to occur (when it 'beds down' to grow and develop), conditions in the womb have to be favourable, too.

Sex – Where, When, How?

Sexual intercourse during a woman's fertile time is essential for conception. Working out your individual fertile time is imperative, but if you prefer not to focus on this, then having lots of sex throughout your cycle will certainly help. Although it's not possible (or necessary) to pinpoint ovulation exactly, a thorough understanding of your own cycle and the signs and symptoms of your most fertile time (as ovulation approaches) can be very beneficial. As mentioned before, aim for lots of sex in the three or four days prior to when ovulation is expected, so the sperm are there, ready and waiting for the egg to appear.

After ovulation, the egg remains in the widest part of the Fallopian tube in anticipation of possible fertilization for up to a maximum of 12 to 24 hours. The whole system is designed to work for you, but being clued up about the basics means you can exploit them to your conceptual advantage.

A Word about Sex Selection

Couples often ask me whether when you have sex affects the baby's gender. While there is some research about this, it is limited and not consistent, and personally I feel that a couple shouldn't restrict their chances of conceiving even further by trying to ensure they have either a boy or a girl. To date there is no reliable evidence to suggest that a baby's gender can be influenced by any natural means such as the timing of intercourse, sexual position or diet.

Case History: Hilary

Hilary, 38, came to see me wanting to conceive again – she already had a son who was 3 years old. I took her through a fertility awareness session and she began regular acupuncture treatments. However, after four months of trying without success Hilary became quite despondent. When I started to dig deeper it became apparent that she really wanted a girl and was limiting when she had sex. She had not discussed this with her husband. At this point I sat her down and gave her a bit of a reality check, outlining that, given her age and fertility cycle, she really did not have the luxury of limiting her chances in this way. She went on to conceive the following month, carried the pregnancy successfully to term and gave birth to a beautiful baby boy.

Whether you have sex at night, in the morning or the middle of the afternoon won't much matter – although, because levels of the male hormone testosterone are higher in the morning, your partner may find it easier to respond to order then!

What Happens Next?

After ejaculation, which moves the sperm into the vagina with some force, the ejaculate begins to coagulate slightly, becoming less watery and more jelly-like. Sperm are already beginning to migrate into the womb and, if assisted by the woman's fertile mucus secretions, will climb efficiently up into the Fallopian tubes. If the egg is still at the top of the Fallopian tube, the tube will stay marginally more open to ease the sperm's passage to the egg.

The tails of the sperm work hard to propel them forward, but it can still take them anything up to two hours to reach the egg because it takes thousands of tail movements to move just 1 centimetre forward. Over the next couple of days, sperm alternately move forward and rest, in order to conserve their energy. Some sperm may rest for a while in the very complex glands that line the cervical canal (neck of the womb) waiting for the egg to be released. It's a boon that healthy sperm can survive for between three and five (and, in rare cases, up to seven) days in a woman's reproductive tract, given that the chances for fertilizing an egg are limited to once per fertile cycle. However, the sperm that actually fertilizes the egg has to be both healthy and vigorous – especially as it can take up to four hours to penetrate the outer covering of the egg!

The stage just prior to the sperm penetrating the egg is an interesting one. At any given time there may be hundreds of sperm swimming around the egg, looking for a way in. The sperm that manages to find an access point usually does so by removing some of the nutrient cells surrounding the egg. Each sperm effectively acts as a drill, but only one can enter as, once one sperm has found a way in, the egg undergoes a chemical change in composition which denies access to any further sperm.

As the sperm passes through the shell of the egg into the cytoplasm, it sheds its protective head, which in turn makes the sperm's genetic material available. It is only now that the male and female cells can merge, producing a new genetic code and the start of a potential life. Within the fertilized egg, the cell divides and continues dividing to produce what is referred to as a blastocyst – an accumulation of cells that have the potential to implant.

The egg is usually fertilized within the Fallopian tube, where it rests in the folds of the protective mucous membrane before beginning its journey down into the womb.

What the fertilized egg needs now is a womb with a nice, thick, blood-rich lining into which it can embed. However, the tiny embryo is, effectively, a foreign body within the mother's system because its protein composition differs from hers. Because of this, the mother's immune system is likely to reject it as it would any other foreign body. This is a precarious time for the embryo; it has to persuade the mother's body not to reject it, but to allow it to latch on to the lining of the womb and continue its development.

Many eggs, even if fertilized successfully, don't embed, for a variety of reasons (see Fertility Work-up chapter). One of the reasons may be this immunological response – the woman's body rejects the embryo. A great deal of research is currently being done on this, especially as for some women it is a recurrent problem that leads to repeated miscarriages and an inability to conceive.

The endometrium, or lining of the womb, is much more than just a bunch of cells. It is very sensitive to the hormone levels circulating in a woman's blood, and it also produces many proteins of its own, many of which are used to nourish the growing embryo. However, the endometrium also contains a lot of immune cells, which have to be persuaded not to reject the tiny embryo.

The Difference between Fertilization and Conception

The fertilization process begins when the quickest sperm penetrates the outer shell of the egg. Within a few minutes of penetrating the egg, the genetic material from the sperm and egg fuse: at this moment a unique genetic code – a human embryo – is created.

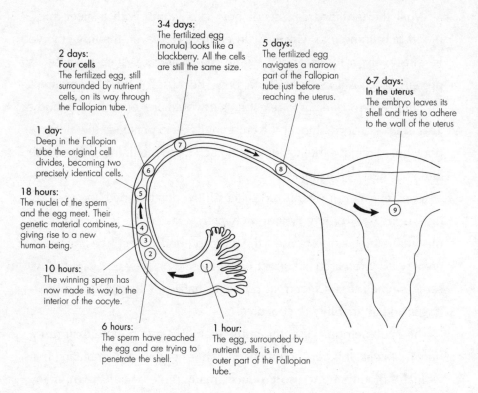

3-4 days:
The fertilized egg (morula) looks like a blackberry. All the cells are still the same size.

2 days:
Four cells
The fertilized egg, still surrounded by nutrient cells, on its way through the Fallopian tube.

5 days:
The fertilized egg navigates a narrow part of the Fallopian tube just before reaching the uterus.

6-7 days:
In the uterus
The embryo leaves its shell and tries to adhere to the wall of the uterus

1 day:
Deep in the Fallopian tube the original cell divides, becoming two precisely identical cells.

18 hours:
The nuclei of the sperm and the egg meet. Their genetic material combines, giving rise to a new human being.

10 hours:
The winning sperm has now made its way to the interior of the oocyte.

6 hours:
The sperm have reached the egg and are trying to penetrate the shell.

1 hour:
The egg, surrounded by nutrient cells, is in the outer part of the Fallopian tube.

On Days 2 to 5, the fertilized egg travels down the Fallopian tube, dividing as it goes: after 48 hours there are four cells, then eight cells, then, by Day 4, it is hard to distinguish individual cells. The fertilized egg, at this point, looks like a tiny blackberry. Another day later the first clear division of tasks among the cells can be detected. At this stage the fertilized egg is referred to medically as a *blastocyst*. Some cells will develop into an embryo, some into the placenta. The last part of the journey for the blastocyst through the narrow end of the Fallopian tube into the uterine cavity takes a few hours. (If the embryo gets stuck here, an ectopic pregnancy will result.)

Just before the blastocyst 'lands' in the womb, it sheds its capsule, selects a spot to settle and begins to imbed (implantation), when the fertilized embryo implants into the lining of the womb. The completion of the process of implantation is conception. This is a delicate time and dependent on the right environment within the womb.

So fertilization can occur without conception, but conception can't occur without fertilization. A woman's egg may be fertilized, but if there is no conception (implantation) then the fertilized egg disintegrates and is lost along with the next menstrual bleed.

On Days 6 to 7 after fertilization, the embryo in the uterus is an 'invader' with a protein composition completely different from and alien to the mother's, and therefore subject to being rejected by her body. Specialized cells in the embryo called *trophoblasts* (which later become the placenta) begin growing in the uterine lining along with immune cells, as communication begins through the mutual exchange of hormones called *cytokines*. If the levels of these cytokines is unbalanced or too high, they can attack the embryo and cause the mother's body to reject it. We'll discuss this and other possible problems in more detail in Part 3 of this book.

part two
preparing your body for pregnancy

the right nutrition

Can I eat this? Should I give up that? These are the kinds of questions I am asked when discussing nutrition with women and their partners when they come to me for help with getting pregnant.

With so many weight-loss diets around, the word 'diet' has become associated with 'good' and 'bad' foods – and we seem to be losing a sense of reality about food. Food is vital. It should provide us with what we need in terms of nutrients. It should be fresh, wholesome, in season and varied to provide the appropriate balance of protein, fats, carbohydrates, vitamins and minerals.

Food is also inextricably linked to digestion. In order to get the best from what you eat, you need to understand your digestive system, and what can prevent it from working well.

A lot of the clients I see do eat a lot of ready-made meals because of their busy lifestyles. These foods are often laden with salt, fats and additives! Many women are also under the illusion that low-fat products and 'diet' products are better for you – they are not! They tend to be full of chemicals and sugar. The latest trend in supermarkets is the 'free from' range, to cater to the allergy market. These products may be free from wheat gluten, dairy, carbs, etc., but when you look more closely they are full of fat and sugar, and glued together with cheap ingredients with no nutritional value at all. No wonder our bodies can have problems processing all of this.

I am always trying to get the message across that my clients should eat foods that are in season and as close to their natural state as possible. That means milk, butter – not margarine, because of its trans-fatty acids – a little cream and cheese. Make an effort to buy fresh produce. Don't do a big supermarket shop once a week; buy fresh veg more often than this. Follow your body: there's a reason why eating salads in winter seems 'not right' – your body craves warming foods at this time of year. Remember, if you want to make changes, you have to plan ahead. It will pay dividends.

The way I work with nutrition is to reinforce the message about balance – not an excess of one item or another – and to use food, rather than supplements, to provide the nutrition you need. I am increasingly seeing couples who are taking up to 20 different vitamin and mineral supplements a day. When I look at the questionnaires they have completed before we meet, it is immediately apparent that they are probably not even absorbing the supplements they take, so they are doing no good at all. Their digestive system is at fault, probably because of the effect not just of the food they are eating, but of their lifestyle – stress, workload, emotional state, etc. Primarily, nutrition is about the food we eat, and how we eat it, not the supplements we take (which can help to make up for deficiencies but are not a substitute for healthy eating).

When you think of what a woman's body has to do each month – balancing hormones, producing an egg, ovulation, enriching the lining of the womb, possible fertilization – then it is unsurprising that her nutritional status is crucial to this, to provide her body with the nourishment it needs. If she is deficient in some way, then the body prioritizes its needs, and reproduction is not a priority when health is compromised. Remember, the body is always trying to achieve balance.

Fertility is a whole-body event, not something that happens just in our reproductive organs. The six principles we work to at our clinic help to restore balance in couples' eating habits and restore or enhance fertility:

a) improving the workings of the digestive system so that it is able to absorb vital nutrients from food

b) restoring blood sugar balance for good hormonal control

c) restoring the acid/alkaline balance in the body (see page 113)

d) assessing the lifestyle changes necessary to ensure that you minimize environmental hormone-disrupters in your life (painkillers, alcohol, cigarettes, drugs, MSG, aspartame) which may be affecting fertility by depleting the body of essential nutrients

e) reducing stress – which has a powerful effect on the digestive system

f) looking at weight.

One immediate effect of assessing and correcting nutritional deficiencies is that any underlying imbalance and associated fertility problems, for example menstrual problems, PCOS (polycystic ovary syndrome) or endometriosis, will benefit immediately as hormonal balance improves following improved nutrition and digestion.

Although we tend to emphasize the importance of nutrition for women, it is of similar importance to men – this an area much neglected when it comes to trying to improve a couple's chances of conceiving. For men, it is easy to improve the health of sperm by eating healthy foods, in conjunction with the appropriate nutritional supplements if necessary, over a four-month period to fit in with the body's natural cycle of sperm production.

The recommendations we offer are based not on faddy diets but on realistic goals, working with a couple to see what foods they like, what their lifestyles are like and what is manageable for them. There 'food fascists', who have come to dominate discussions about nutrition, have led women in particular to give up nearly every food. We recommend the 80/20 rule – being health-conscious about what you eat 80 per cent of the time. Even when you 'relax', give yourself quality: if you have chocolate, have a small piece of really good chocolate; if you have a glass of wine, have one glass of a really nice wine.

Couples have so often stopped being good to themselves when trying for a baby. Food is a pleasurable experience; it enhances mood and releases endorphins. Many women I see are on very restrictive diets for long periods of time, and feel they have lost all pleasure or enjoyment in food. There is nothing more depressing than eating boring foods, and research has shown that eliminating so many foods from your diet, especially carbs, can leave you feeling depressed.

A First Step

My recommendation is that every couple about to embark on pregnancy should detox first! This means giving your system a rest for a short period of time – say about 10 days. Effectively this provides a clean state from which to progress. So often the body is having to deal with a toxic overload from a poor diet, excess alcohol, cigarette smoking, or a badly functioning gut, that it makes no sense even to start a programme of fertility-promotion without it. This applies equally to men as to women, as their sperm benefit hugely from reviewing their lifestyle and cleaning up their diet. Starting with a detox is the most positive first step any couple can take.

Kicking off with a good detox (see page 141) is a hugely beneficial start to improve your overall health – but remember, a good detox is not just a nutritional detox, it's a physical and emotional detox as well, where you chuck out old habits and allow new, healthier ones to take their place.

Toxic Load

Food production today includes a huge range of chemicals, preservatives and additives in its processing: from antibiotics and hormones in meat production, to the hydrogenation of fats (which produce free radicals) and the use of pesticides, chemical preservatives, flavourings and colourings including MSG (mono-sodium glutamate, used as a 'flavour-enhancer') and aspartame (an artificial sweetener found widely in diet sodas, etc.). While considered safe in isolation by the authorities, consider how large a part they play in your daily diet. The burden soon adds up, and places an extra strain on the body's ability to process and detoxify. While the body's capacity for processing and eliminating all these additional chemicals is good, it will concentrate on what is crucial for existence, leaving less energy and ability to function properly in less crucial areas – such as hormonal balance. Your aim, in choosing what you eat and drink, is to reduce the burden on your body, allowing it to function well in its main systems – reproductive, circulatory, endocrine, nervous – and in optimum health, making conception more possible.

Aspartame and MSG

Aspartame is an additive found in diet drinks, chewing gums and sugar-substitute products. In the digestive system, aspartame breaks down to formaldehyde – this is what scientists use to preserve specimens, so imagine what it can do to your system. It is believed to accumulate in the cells, causing damage to the cell DNA.

MSG (monosodium glutamate) is a very common flavour-enhancer used in foods. It has been found to cause infertility in test animals. There are many, many products that include MSG. It is found in gelatine, textured protein products, yeast extract and many other foods. Other products that often contain MSG include bouillons and broths, soy sauce, seasonings and anything fermented. Also check labels for 'pea protein', 'whey protein' and 'corn protein' – these are just new terms for 'hydrolysed' peas/whey/corn, etc., and the hydrolysing process always includes MSG.

So choose organic products when you can, grown in season. Strawberries in January mean they may well be genetically modified, have been exposed to pesticides, picked before fully ripe, shipped and stored – their nutritional value to you is virtually nil by the time they arrive on your table, so don't waste your money. Fruit and vegetables that are fresh, even if not organic, are better – try your local farmers' markets, or buy daily rather than in bulk. We are very wedded to super-market shopping these days, which is partly a lifestyle choice and also linked to the excessively hectic pace of modern life. Try to change your shopping habits when you can – taking 10 minutes to pick up the things you know you need at a nearby shop on your way home every day or so certainly beats spending the whole of every Saturday morning at the megastore on the edge of town.

Of course, I understand that not everyone can afford to eat organically. It is still expensive and in my experience some organic produce is not always even that good. The point is, don't get bogged down or let this become another source of stress: so many couples I see are worried that if their diet is not 100 per cent organic, like all the books say it should be, they won't get pregnant. As mentioned earlier, just try to eat foods as close to their natural source as possible, in season and without additives.

Slow Down!

All of us tend to eat too much, too fast. 'Fast food' refers almost as much to the speed at which we eat as to the speed with which we prepare it – or heat it up in the microwave. Eating quickly and not chewing properly results in food passing too quickly through the digestive system, without providing its full nutritional benefit, and this leaves us feeling hungry and hence eating more. Eating slowly satisfies the digestive system, and our appetites, better. Try it – you'll probably find yourself eating less.

In addition, we tend to eat when we are tired, stressed and anxious – food has lost its social and pleasurable capacity for many and become just another thing to be scheduled into a busy day. A stressed, anxious and tired digestive system functions poorly, making what we eat less nutritionally accessible. When it comes to considering our fertility and health, there are extremely good arguments for almost all of us to reassess how our eating habits fit into our lifestyles.

The ancient Chinese believe that certain organs work over a 24-hour cycle, and this is a feature of Traditional Chinese Medicine to which I subscribe, because I have seen the benefits of this approach. The peak time for the stomach's ability to function is between 7 and 9 a.m., and the resting time for the stomach is between 7 and 9 p.m. So the optimum time for our most nutritious and digestively demanding meal of the day is in the morning, when the system is fully rested, empty and functioning at its best.

The old saying – breakfast like a king, lunch like a prince, dine like a pauper – was rooted in the knowledge that breakfast is the most important meal of the day when it comes to digestion. Eating a large meal late at night, which gets the digestive juices all revved up and is very stimulating for the body, inevitably makes sleep difficult. More importantly, because the stomach isn't working to its optimum capacity, the digestive process is slower, so we can't benefit fully from the nutritional content of the food we eat. And because the evening is the beginning of the rest period for the stomach, food remains undigested and fermentation can occur as a result.

Foods eaten raw, like fruit and vegetables, have a greater propensity for fermentation. Fermentation in itself isn't bad, the body can cope with it – it's a process that occurs naturally in the gut with alcohols, sugars, yeasts, etc. – but eat fruit or raw foods early on in the day, so the body has time to digest them properly.

The Chinese classification of foods into yin and yang has a contemporary equivalent in the acid/alkaline balance and the hot/cold balance of the foods we eat today.

Traditional Chinese Medicine and Your Diet

The ancient Chinese had very good guidelines about food and diet that fit very much in with what you should be aiming for. Balancing yin and yang (that is, acid and alkaline) foods, and eating foods as they are available in season will have many benefits for couples trying to conceive.

TCM recognizes food as the main source of energy. Each organ has an impact and a different way of using the foods we eat, and each food has different energetic qualities. Hot foods are more yang in quality. It is always yang foods, which are warming foods, which I try to encourage women to take when trying for a baby. Too many women today eat too many cold, raw foods, which use a lot more of the body's energy and are harder to digest. Some foods in Chinese medicine build up the blood; other foods help to draw heat and dampness from the body. The different tastes of foods are considered important for the body's balance as well. The five tastes are classified as sweet, spicy, sour, bitter and salty, and a good meal should include all of the flavours. Having one of these flavours in excess creates imbalance in the body. For example, eating too many sweet things adversely affects the spleen. Too many salty things affect the kidneys. I see a lot of women who have a high salt intake and raised FSH levels. So food in Chinese medicine is calculated to supply all of our organs with different balanced tastes and energetic qualities for good health.

Kidney Foods – 'The Crown Jewels'

In TCM, the kidney meridian is very important for hormone balance, fertility and reproduction, not least because the kidneys are believed to balance all the yin and yang in the body, govern sperm production, and regulate the hormonal production of the menstrual cycle. The kidneys store our *yin*, which is our vital essence, as well as the genetic material RNA and DNA. It is necessary for both of these to be in good supply for a man and woman to be able to conceive. So in Chinese nutrition there are foods that build the kidneys and strengthen our genetic material. These foods are:

- Bee pollen and Royal Jelly (as long as you are not allergic to pollen)
- Blue-green algae, which contains chlorophyll
- Spirulina, rich in nutrients
- Foods high in essential fatty acids (EFAs), especially DHA
- Nuts and seeds.

Another feature of the traditional Chinese approach is the value of effective, regular detoxing (see page 141).

Digestion

It's important to remember that our hormones are made from the foods we eat. You can be taking every nutritional supplement under the sun and eating the purest organic food, but if your digestive system is weak you will not be absorbing the nutrients you need.

Hormonal Health and the Digestive System

Every week I see couples who are not really considering what they are eating in relation to their fertility problems. They take supplements to compensate for a deficient diet, not to enhance a good one. Food should always be your first source of nutrition. Any digestive system already trying to cope with an excess of additives, pesticides, hormonal and environmental factors loses some of its capacity to digest food properly. All the supplements in the world won't compensate for this. You wouldn't consider putting leaded petrol or diesel in a lead-free car, because it isn't designed to run on that fuel. The same is true of the body. Poor fuel means our bodies cannot function properly. What's more, poor fuel – in the form of the rubbish we often eat – means that the body's energy is taken up with dealing with toxins rather than doing the job it was designed for – which, in the case of the couples I see, is trying to conceive.

A poor diet and a poor digestive system put the body into hormonal havoc, forcing it to deal with crisis after crisis, and putting it out of balance. The effort required by the body to break down, eliminate and rebalance the body when it's exposed to continuous poor eating habits is enormous. The result is that the body draws on its reserves of valuable nutrients which should be available to balance your energy, mood, hormonal cycle and blood sugar levels. Busy with all that, you may as well forget fertility – it is no longer the body's priority.

Do you suffer from any of the following?
- constipation?
- diarrhoea?
- bloating?
- flatulence?
- bad breath?
- stomach pains?
- indigestion?
- a burning sensation in your stomach?
- food intolerances or allergies?

If you experience several of these, chances are you have a digestive problem. Many of us do.

Fortunately, the body responds extremely well once changes have been made to help restore its internal balance. Reviewing not just what you eat, but how you eat it and when, all play a part. For many this can feel like quite a dramatic lifestyle change but, once made, the rewards in general health and vitality – and the achieving of a pregnancy – make it well worth the effort.

The Digestive Tract

Good digestion starts in the mouth – always make sure you chew your food properly! The stomach, only the size of a fist, receives the chewed food where it is mixed with a variety of digestive juices. Eating under pressure – on the run, when you are angry, frustrated or stressed – will weaken your digestion.

The small intestine is also crucially important for the immune system. A large percentage of immune cells are made here, so the function of the small intestine is integral to a strong immune system. The small intestine is lined with thousands of small finger-like projections, called *villi*, where the liquefied food we have eaten comes into extremely close proximity to blood capillaries and where the absorption of nutrients takes place. If food passes through the small intestine too quickly, or if there is any sort of tension or spasm that reduces the blood supply to this area during this crucial process, then the absorption of nutrients is inhibited.

On a recent visit to the Mayr Clinic in Austria, where they believe that all problems in the body come down to problems in the digestive system, I discovered that their professional principles, like mine, are based very much on ancient Chinese philosophy when it comes to nutrition and diet. The Mayr Clinic believes very much in going back to basics: chewing your food well to utilize the digestive juices in the saliva and to stimulate the digestive juices in the stomach in preparation for the food's arrival there. While breakfast and lunch are served at the clinic, there is no evening meal. Food is taken when the digestive system is best able to digest it.

Back to Basics

So – without stressing yourself out about this – try to incorporate the following basic changes gently into your diet over a few weeks or months:

a) Eat only when you are hungry.

b) Chew your food well.

c) Make time to eat, don't eat on the run.

d) Don't drink water before you eat, as this dilutes the stomach's digestive juices.

e) Don't eat if you are angry, emotional, upset or tired – in Chinese philosophy this is believed to knot your *qi* and block digestion.

f) Avoid raw foods late in the evening, as these are hard to digest and use up a lot of energy in doing so – if you want to include salads or juice in your diet, do so in the morning when digestion is better.

g) Avoid raw juices late in the evening, or take them only first thing in the morning so you give your system enough time to digest them properly.

h) Limit carbohydrates after 4 p.m., as they can cause fermentation. The digestive system slows down later in the day, and certain foods eaten at this time will ferment in the gut and give off alcohols, which can weaken the digestive system.

i) Eat only until full, don't overeat – and remember your stomach is only the size of a balled fist.

j) Aim to have a larger meal at lunchtime than in the evening as often as you can.

k) Aim for a 20 per cent acid, 80 per cent alkaline balance (see page 115).

l) Use natural products like butter, milk, cream rather than low-fat products, which have chemicals added. Margarine is a hydrogenated fat product which creates free radicals (more about these later).

m) No fruit after lunch.

n) No refined sugars.

o) Cut back on wheat consumption.

p) Cut back on tea, coffee and alcohol consumption.

q) Drink lots of water, preferably filtered, but not at mealtimes.

r) Eat small amounts of protein, and lots of lightly cooked vegetables.

This is quite a comprehensive list and, for many couples who come to see me, represents an enormous change. Start by integrating those items on the list that come easily, and build towards the full list, which will do a great deal to help make the digestive changes needed.

Common Digestive Problems

Dysbiosis or abnormal gut fermentation (Candida)

Candida has become a buzz word; I see too many clients on far too restrictive diets, and they're miserable as a result.

There are many symptoms associated with this condition, and often there is not an obvious pattern of symptoms. The most common are irritable bowel-type symptoms such as bloating and flatulence. However, classic allergic symptoms such as rhinitis (constantly runny nose), asthma and urticaria (skin rash) may also be part of the picture.

Abnormal gut fermentation can also lead to a deficiency in B vitamins, zinc and magnesium.

Dietary Strategy for Dysbiosis

People with dysbiosis commonly have marked cravings for sugars and yeasty foods. Those with an apparent intolerance to sugars, starches, yeast and cheese may not experience intolerance symptoms but abnormal gut fermentation instead. These people often show a dramatic response to a diet low in yeasty, mould-containing and fermentable foods, whether or not they are taking anti-fungal medication. After some months of careful adherence to the regime, many people become able to manage the condition themselves.

Foods to Include

- Eat a wholefood diet consisting of wholegrains such as brown rice, millet, quinoa and buckwheat, fresh vegetables, beans and pulses, fish and free-range eggs.
- Eat wholegrain breads such as rye and wholewheat as long as they are yeast free.
- Use cold-pressed extra virgin olive oil on vegetables and salads.
- Limit cheese to once or twice a week only and have fresh hard cheeses like Parmesan.
- Use a little organic unsalted butter.
- Replace milk with almond, rice or oat milk.
- Balance blood sugar levels by reducing carbohydrates and introducing protein with every meal.
- Eat lots of garlic and live natural organic yoghurt.

Foods to Avoid

- Sugar and sweeteners – confectionery and preserves – desserts and puddings
- Fruit – dried or crystallized fruit – glacé fruit – fruit tinned in syrup – grapes, melon, over-ripe, damaged or mouldy fruit (especially soft fruit)
- Cereals and grains (bread, biscuits and cakes), yeasts, all breakfast cereals containing sugar, and/or dried fruit and nuts – all breads except unleavened bread/bread made without yeast
- Milk and milk products – unpasteurized milk – cottage cheese, cream cheese – processed cheese – blue cheeses – cheese with mouldy skin, e.g. Brie – any cheese covered in mould
- Processed meats such as ham and salami
- Vegetables that are naturally sweet and have a high glycaemic index (sweet potatoes, baked potatoes, cooked carrots) – pre-prepared salads with dressings – ordinary baked beans
- Soups, sauces and condiments – tinned and packet soups – pickles and chutneys
- Stimulants such as spices, tea, coffee and alcohol
- Beverages – all fruit juices – ordinary fizzy drinks and fruit squashes – flavoured mineral waters, all beer, wine, cider, sherry and port

Friendly Bacteria

Gut bacteria play a major role in health generally, and in hormone metabolism particularly. An overgrowth of undesirable bacteria will lead to the reabsorption of toxins back into the bloodstream from the bowel. Healthy gut bacteria provide a defence against the toxic patho-genic bacteria that can cause many health problems. The *Lactobacillus acidophilus* bacteria found in live or bio-yoghurts are protective, as well as promoting the excretion of 'old' oestrogens in the faeces. You may be advised to take a concentrated supplement to re-colonize your gut bacteria initially, particularly if you have taken antibiotics or the Pill in the recent past.

Foods that provide fuel for good bacteria include onions and artichokes.

Constipation

I am including constipation in this chapter because it affects so many people and is so closely related to diet. Many of the women I see think that it is OK to have a bowel movement every three to four days – or for some just once a week. It is important that you eat plenty of fibre (up to 25g a day, but no more than this) contained in wholegrains, fruits and vegetables. Fibre binds to metabolized hormones, toxins, pesticides and chemicals that can be damaging to your health, making it easier for you to excrete them efficiently.

Linseeds are a particularly beneficial form of fibre, plus being high in omega-3 essential fatty acids. With water, they will swell up in your digestive tract, forming a bulky stool, which will pass along the bowel quickly and efficiently. Linseeds and water also produce a mucilaginous substance, as you will notice when you soak them. This is very soothing and protective and aids the passage of the stool.

You should also aim to drink at least 1½ litres of filtered water a day.

Foods to Avoid

- Refined processed foods
- Sweet sugary foods
- Cooked cheese
- Dairy products
- Fizzy drinks
- Too much meat
- Tea

Foods to Eat

- Oats and oat bran
- Beans, pulses and lentils
- Whole grains – brown rice and grainy wheat-free breads
- Buckwheat
- Corn on the cob
- Cauliflower
- Apples
- Pears
- Green leafy vegetables, root vegetables, broccoli stalks
- Prunes
- Cherries
- Figs
- Kiwi fruit
- Psyllium husks
- At least 1.5 litres of filtered water a day

What Else Helps?

Gentle exercise is very helpful in avoiding constipation – try walking, Pilates, yoga, swimming and rebounding (though the last in this list should *not* be undertaken if you might be pregnant).

Poor posture is also a factor in constipation, as the abdominal organs can become compressed, reducing blood flow. Try the Alexander Technique or yoga. Osteopathy (particularly visceral osteopathy) is useful in cases of chronic or recurrent constipation. Taking time when you feel the need for a bowel movement, and feeling relaxed in a warm, comfortable environment can help immensely.

Food Allergies and Intolerances

An allergy is a very specific response which involves the release of immune-system antibodies (IgE). These are released in response to proteins in foods (such as milk) and trigger the release of histamines, which cause itching and inflammation. It is almost always an immediate or very quick reaction.

A food intolerance does not cause this effect, though the symptoms can be almost as unpleasant as those of a full-blown allergy. In either case, however, I believe that building up your digestive system can improve symptoms.

Dairy and Wheat

I am often asked, 'How much dairy or wheat should I include in my diet?' Many people comment on how much better they feel when they cut these out of their diets: headaches, bloating and symptoms of irritable bowel all seem to disappear. I do find it hard to believe, however, that everyone has a wheat or dairy allergy, though I do agree that most of us do eat these foods too frequently.

If you feel you have a problem with dairy foods, cut them out for a couple of weeks (you can switch to goat's milk or sheep's milk products instead) and see how you feel. Having said this, organic milk tends not to pose problems, and I believe in the health benefits of whole milk, butter, cream and cheeses (not semi-skimmed or skimmed), as these help the body to make the best use of fat-soluble vitamins. I am also loath to recommend large amounts of soya milk, as it has an effect on female hormones and male fertility.

The approach you take to wheat should be similar. Switch to rye and oat biscuits, corn pasta and other wheat-free products and see how you feel. After a month or so, reintroduce wheat breads or pastas but only twice a week. It may be that you have just been having too much wheat, and that cutting back a bit is all you need to feel better.

Caffeine

As mentioned elsewhere in this book, caffeine is dehydrating and a stimulant. I always ask clients to give up coffee and other drinks and foods that contain caffeine. This substance can increase the time it takes to conceive and has been linked to miscarriage and premature birth. It is best to cut it out if you can, or just save it as a very occasional treat. Remember, though, to cut it out slowly, as you will experience withdrawal symptoms (headaches, for example) if you are used to drinking a lot of coffee, tea and colas and suddenly go 'cold turkey'.

Balancing Your Blood Sugar Levels

- Do you need something to get you going in the morning?
- Do you have tea, coffee and/or cola regularly?
- Do you crave sweet things?
- Do you feel drowsy during the day?
- Are you unusually hungry?
- Do you pass water regularly?

It is important to avoid fluctuation in blood sugar levels, because low blood sugar can cause many unwanted symptoms like headaches, dizziness, tiredness, lack of energy, irritability, cravings for sweet things and PMS. Sugary drinks and foods, and refined, processed carbohydrates are digested very quickly, causing a rapid increase in the glucose in your bloodstream. High glucose levels are undesirable, and so insulin is released in order to lower blood sugar levels in the blood. This can lead to hypoglycaemia (low blood sugar) and the feelings of tiredness and irritability mentioned above. This is also when the cravings for sweet foods occur and the whole cycle begins again. Stimulants like coffee, tea and alcohol also have the same effect.

Refined carbohydrates contain no valuable nutrients and will cause you to gain weight, and excess weight exacerbates hormone imbalances. Continually yo-yoing blood sugar levels eventually exhaust the pancreas, where insulin is produced, and then hyperglycaemia (high blood sugar) is the result. This has major long-term health implications such as diabetes and cardiovascular disease.

Hormone production and fertility are also affected, because oestrogen is produced from fat cells – the more fat cells, the more oestrogen. Excess weight can create an excess of oestrogen, which will disturb your hormonal balance, especially with regard to progesterone. Progesterone rises when oestrogen levels drop after ovulation, and is responsible for helping conception, implantation and the thickening of the womb lining necessary for the initial stability and growth of the embryo. If oestrogen levels stay high, then there is no stimulus for the secretion of progesterone, which is so essential for pregnancy to occur and progress.

Another feature of yo-yoing blood sugar levels is that, when they drop, adrenaline is released – and this also interferes with hormone production. Adrenaline and cortisol secretion at elevated levels in response to continuous stress has a comparable effect on hormone production. And if you take into consideration the effect stress also has on our eating and drinking habits, then the combination of this and disordered blood sugar levels can have profound effects on fertility.

Eating little and often of good, wholesome and nutritious foods won't make you fat. Your metabolism will function properly, you will have more energy, and you will no longer have cravings for sweet, refined foods.

a) Eat regularly.

b) Always have breakfast.

c) Always mix proteins and carbohydrates together in a meal, as this delays the digestive process, giving a gradual slow release of glucose into the bloodstream.

d) Eat complex carbohydrates – wholemeal bread and pasta, oats, potatoes.

e) Eat fresh fruits and lightly cooked fresh vegetables.

f) Cut out refined carbohydrates – sugary cakes, biscuits and sweets, soft drinks, white bread, white rice and pasta.

g) Snack on nuts – particularly almonds, Brazil nuts, macadamia nuts and unsalted cashews – and on pumpkin, sunflower and sesame seeds.

h) Eat beans – butter beans, kidney beans, chickpeas and lentils – which combine carbohydrate and protein to reduce yo-yoing blood sugar levels.

The good news is, once your blood sugar is balanced you won't feel the need to snack in between meals.

Cortisol Deficiency: Stress Exhaustion

When first stressed, the adrenal glands produce up to 40 hormones including adrenaline and cortisol, boost blood sugar levels and also release DHEA. DHEA helps increase energy levels and our resistance to stress; as stress continues, however, cortisol levels will tend to go up and DHEA levels will fall. If stress becomes chronic, the adrenal glands become exhausted and can no longer help the body deal with stress.

Cortisol has numerous important roles in the body including regulating the way the body uses proteins, fats and carbohydrates. Over time, the body's continuous demands made for stress hormones can no longer be met – and the levels of cortisol required by the body become deficient.

Although cortisol isn't a fertility hormone, it plays a crucial role in the interplay between the body's hormones, and can affect the balance of the fertility hormones because it is circulated in the body by a protein known as CBG (cortisol-binding globulin), which also carries progesterone.

The two most noticeable affects of cortisol deficiency are debilitating tiredness and unstable blood sugar, and the two main causes are long-term low-level stress and poor nutrition. We think we can persistently work 18 hours a day, exist on junk food and forgo real relaxation to recuperate – but our bodies tell a different story.

The main solutions for cortisol deficiency are usually the implementation of what are, for some people, major lifestyle changes. A reduction of stimulants such as sugar, cigarettes, caffeine and alcohol means a comprehensive change, while a healthy diet with a good balance of nutrients needs to be introduced. Finally, where there are signs of cortisol deficiency affecting hormone balance and inhibiting conception, learning relaxation techniques (see page 184) – and using them daily – is essential.

The Glycaemic Index (GI)

Researchers have created a scale from 1-100 called the Glycaemic Index. This is based on how quickly a food is digested, metabolized and then released into the bloodstream as glucose. This scale was originally designed to help people with diabetes maintain controlled blood sugar levels. However, it is also useful for general health purposes, too, as foods that have a low or moderate GI ranking make us feel full for longer, providing constant stable blood sugar and reducing the associated symptoms of fluctuating blood sugar levels.

Glucose is ranked as 100 as it is absorbed most quickly, giving fast release and short-term energy. Foods ranked this high are best avoided altogether, or otherwise mixed with a little protein or fat, which slows down glucose release.

The way that certain foods are cooked also affects their GI ranking. For example, boiled potatoes have a medium GI index, while mashed and baked potatoes are high. White rice is high, while basmati rice is medium. Foods with a low GI ranking also include those that are higher in soluble fibre – most fruits and vegetables, wholegrains such as oats, lentils and other pulses. Foods on the lower end of the GI scale raise blood sugar more slowly and are consequently the ones that will make you feel fuller and satisfied for longer.

Low GI Foods
Foods ranking 40 or under on the index include:
- Apples, plums, pears, dried apricots, peaches, cherries
- All pulses – lentils, kidney beans, baked beans, cannelloni beans, flageolet beans, butter beans, chickpeas
- Green leafy vegetables – broccoli, Brussels sprouts, cabbage, mangetout, leeks, green beans
- Cauliflower, mushrooms, avocados, courgettes, peppers

- Whole grains, wholegrain rye bread, oats
- Yoghurt
- Nuts and seeds

Medium GI Foods

Foods ranking between 40 and 60 on the index, which should only be eaten in moderate amounts, include:

- Grapes, under-ripe bananas, mangoes, figs, kiwi fruit
- Sweet corn, peas, raw carrots, beetroot, boiled potatoes, sweet potatoes
- Oat biscuits, popcorn, whole-wheat pasta, wholemeal bread, brown basmati rice

High GI Foods

Foods ranking over 60 on the index should only be eaten in moderation with protein and fat. Avoid completely refined, processed foods, and those with added sweeteners and sugars.

- Baked potatoes, mashed potatoes
- White bread, white rice, white pasta
- Honey, sugar, jam, sweets and chocolate
- Cooked carrots, parsnips, swedes, squash
- Ripe bananas, watermelon, raisins
- Sugared breakfast cereal
- Rice cakes, cous cous

The Acid/Alkaline Balance

In order for the body to function properly, there needs to be a balance (yes, there's that word again!) of acid and alkaline foods in the diet. Acidity and alkalinity are measured by what is called pH. The pH scale is between 1 and 14, with any measurement below 7 indicating acidity. The 'normal' pH level that is considered healthy is 7.4. Each calibration on the pH scale is 10 times the previous one, so, for example, if your pH level is 6.4 rather than 7.4, it is 10 times more acidic than normal.

Many adults have a pH reading – from saliva, urine or blood – of below this pH norm. For good health – and this includes avoiding other health problems like arthritis, heart disease, osteoporosis, cancer (cancer cells find it hard to exist in an alkaline environment) and kidney disease – keeping the body in an alkaline state is very important.

Through my work at my clinic, and having seen thousands of couples trying to get pregnant over the years, I have become convinced that many of the male/female health problems I see are caused by over-acidity in the body. For some couples, the levels of acidity in their bodies are just too high, making getting pregnant more difficult.

High acid is also caused by stress, and by eating when you are angry or upset. The body needs to be alkaline, and the same is true for the cervical secretions a woman produces each month to enable the sperm to swim to reach the egg. The environment the sperm is in also needs to be alkaline. Anecdotally, a lot of the men we see, who are on high-protein diets, have terrible sperm counts. Also for women on high-protein diets, research shows that high acidity in the uterus stops implantation from taking place. For those of you who are gardeners, you would never dream of trying to sow a seed if the pH of the soil wasn't right. If the soil is not right, the seed cannot grow.

To balance the soil and get the pH right you have to make the necessary lifestyle changes. The ancient Chinese always said that if the soil is well prepared the harvest will be bountiful.

What the body needs for balance

For the body to function properly, its basic state needs to be alkaline, and this is crucial for fertility. The increased female cervical secretions around the time of ovulation need to be alkaline to protect the sperm from the normally acid environment of the vagina. The acid/alkaline balance needs to be 20/80 for optimum functioning, but our typical Westernized diet generally tends to be more acid.

There is another aspect of our generally poor diet that has an effect both on the acid/alkaline balance of the body and on fertility. Typically, the Western diet includes many excess oestrogens, and this is aggravated by a poor diet high in refined sugars and by a weak digestive system, causing permanently raised oestrogen levels.

When oestrogen levels are permanently raised, the body no longer responds to them as it should.

Excess oestrogen in the muscles and circulatory system is converted to acidic waste, further increasing the body's acidity. It's a vicious circle.

If the uterus becomes highly acidic, implantation of a fertilized egg is unlikely. When oestrogen levels are permanently elevated, they no longer react to the body's needs.

Many women experience symptoms of this hormonal imbalance. Heavy periods, endometriosis and PMS, for example, are all clear indicators of hormonal imbalances. What has not been fully appreciated before is how much the food we eat and the poor functioning of our digestive systems affect the balance of our hormones.

Nor is it just a question of eating a balanced diet; it's about ensuring that what you eat and how you eat it create the maximum benefit, allowing full functioning of all the body's systems and allowing the reproductive system a chance to function at a level where sperm production, ovulation, fertilization and conception are possible.

Improving Alkalinity

To improve the situation, it is essential to get back to an alkaline state. We all eat far too many acidic foods. Weight-loss diets based on this ratio are catastrophically bad for both men and women when it comes to trying to get pregnant.

The acid/alkaline balance is easier to maintain than it is to correct, so it's well worth thinking about the dietary changes that need to be made in the long term, as well as in the short term. Keeping in mind the range of foods that fall into the acid/alkaline categories is helpful when making food choices.

Carbonated drinks are worth a special mention, because they also contain high sugar levels and have a pH of around 2.8 – highly acidic. Cut them out immediately as they are so detrimental to your health.

In addition, as the body tries to normalize a highly acidic state, calcium is leached from the bones, creating a potential weakness there and depleting the body further of critical nutrients.

For the cells of any system in the body to function properly, the outside of the cells requires an alkaline environment. The lymphatic system of the body, crucial for maintaining a healthy, detoxed, internal state, functions best in an alkaline environment. The lymphatic system has around 600 to 700 lymph glands, and as much circulating fluid as the blood system, and works extremely hard to support the immune system by removing toxic and acidic waste from body cells, and transporting it to the liver for neutralization and excretion. This is a much-neglected feature of the body's ability to detox, which can benefit greatly from manual lymphatic drainage (MLD – see page 145) – part of the programme I offer my clients.

Getting back to a good acid/alkaline balance of 20/80 per cent is essential for both partners in achieving pregnancy.

80%	**ALKALI AND ACID FOODS**				20%	
EAT IN ABUNDANCE			EAT FREQUENTLY		EAT MODERATELY	
High alkali	Medium alkali	Low alkali	Neutral	Low acid	Medium acid	High acid
Melon	Sweet	Cherries	Cranberries	Blueberries	Sharp	Beef
Lemons	apples	Peaches	Unsalted		mature	(organic)
Limes	Apricots	Oranges	butter	Sunflower	cheese	Chicken
Mango	Avocados	Raspberries	Milk (organic,	seeds		(organic)
Dates	Bananas	Strawberries	natural,	Pumpkin	Whole eggs	Turkey
Figs	Grapefruit	Beetroot	live/bio)	seeds		(organic)
Papaya	Kiwis	Broccoli		Brazil nuts	Fish	Lamb
Grapes	Nectarines	Brussels	Nut & seed	Macadamia	Shellfish	(organic)
	Passion fruit	sprouts	oils (except	nuts		
Kelp &	Pears	Cauliflower	olive)	Walnuts	Wheatgerm	Refined
seaweeds	Tangerines	Artichokes		Cashews	Oats	pasta
	Raisins	Chicory			Rice	
Parsley	Pineapple	Sweetcorn		Cheese	(brown	
Watercress		Cucumber		(except	Basmati)	
	Asparagus	Aubergine		mature/		
Wheatgrass	Carrots	Ginger		sharp)	High-quality	
juice	Celery	Kale			organic	
	Swiss chard	Leeks		Rye	wine	
	Pumpkin	Spring				
	Spinach	onions		Pulses	High-quality	
	Dandelion	Parsnips		Lentils	organic	
	greens	Peppers			coffee	
	Salad leaves	Potatoes with				
	Butternut	skins				
	squash	Sweet				
	Courgettes	tomatoes				
	Pumpkin					
	Peas	Most herbs				
	Green	Curry spices				
	beans					
	Alfalfa	Amaranth				
	sprouts	Millet				
	Garlic	Quinoa				
	Chives					
	Margoram	Almonds				
		Sesame				
	Most	seeds				
	vegetable					
	juices	Olive oil				
		Mayonnaise				
		Tamari				
		Apple cider				
		vinegar				
		Egg yolks				
		Goat's milk				
		Tofu				

Acidity

The most important thing to understand is that all metabolism – of proteins, fats and carbohydrates – produces acidity. Protein, for example, produces sulphuric and phosphoric acids, while fats produce acetic and lactic acid. These acids need to be eliminated from the body as quickly as possible but, in order to prevent damage to the excretory organs (and the kidneys in particular), they have to be neutralized by minerals like calcium, magnesium and potassium. If there are inadequate neutralizing minerals in the diet, the body will use its reserves – in the case of calcium, this involves leaching it from where it is stored in our bones.

Foods that are strongly alkaline, like leafy green vegetables such as broccoli, are high in sodium, potassium, calcium, magnesium, and iron – all of which work to neutralize the acid substances in the body before elimination. (This is one reason why high-protein/low-carb diets don't work long term: Excessive phosphate levels in meats can remove calcium and magnesium from the body.) Keeping the body in a good, balanced, alkaline state avoids the need to deplete the body's reserves of essential minerals. As ever, balance is key – too high an alkaline diet can be detrimental, too.

You will still be eating protein (fish, chicken, dairy, nuts and grains) in small amounts, but these will be balanced by lots of vegetables and fruits, seeds and water. For example, if you eat a piece of (lean, organic) chicken, which is acidic, you can easily balance this by eating a piece of melon (particularly watermelon), which is very alkaline. Another means of creating balance would be to eat a small portion of red meat (again, lean and organic) with lots of vegetables. You can add chicken, fish or beans to salads or to a variety of steamed or stir-fried vegetables, and use tomato sauces with herbs and spices instead of creamy ones. Start the day with hot water and the juice of half a lemon, or include some apple cider vinegar in warm water before meals.

An added benefit is that fruits and vegetables also contain an abundance of immune-enhancing plant chemicals.

Acidic foods to include in your diet could include fresh fish, organic chicken, nuts, seeds, pulses, oats, rye and egg yolks. As far as dairy products go, eat cheese very sparingly, and have a little unsalted butter and plain live organic yoghurt. Have a little bit of honey but in moderation; it *is* alkaline, but also raises blood sugar.

As pesticides and fungicides are acidic, try to buy as much organic produce as you can, but don't worry too much. And remember to wash all fruits and vegetables carefully.

Food Types

Proteins

While you need a regular supply of good protein, especially for cell production (and this includes sperm and eggs), by and large we all have more than is sufficient to meet our needs. And, because protein consists mainly of highly acidic foods, having a diet too high in protein can create problems, as we have seen.

Protein provides amino acids, which are the building-blocks of cells (and this includes hormones, too). We get proteins not only from meat and fish, which are considered primary sources (that is, they contain a full range of amino acids) but also from dairy sources and vegetable sources such as pulses, beans and lentils. Red meat is more acidic than fish or chicken, so we should eat red meat only occasionally (no more than once a week). In terms of how much protein we need per day, 50g is sufficient, and should make up about 15 per cent of your daily calories.

Proteins cooked at high temperatures, especially barbecued foods, also produce by-products that can damage cells' DNA.

Too low a protein intake, which can sometimes occur in vegans and vegetarians, can also be detrimental. If you are not getting enough protein you may also become deficient in vitamins B_2 and B_6, which are needed to neutralize acidity. A diet too low in protein can also depress the GNRH (gonadotrophin-releasing hormone) level, responsible for the release of FSH (follicle-stimulating hormone) and LH (luteinizing hormone). Protein is crucial to sperm production and, in fact, to our libidos.

It's easy to see why weight-loss diets that rely on a high-protein, low-carbohydrate mix can be so detrimental to health. A diet that relies heavily on a high protein intake will take the body into an acidic state, which over a period of time can be damaging. The body will always try to regain balance, and if this means depleting stores of alkaline minerals, by leaching calcium from the bones, it will. What is OK in the short term becomes damaging to the body in the long term.

Protein is essential for growth and repair, and ensuring adequate amounts is essential when you are trying to conceive naturally or prior to IVF to ensure the development of the embryo. However, high amounts of protein are not a good idea, as there appears to be some evidence suggesting that the ammonia produced as by-product of excessive protein metabolism may interfere in some way with embryo implantation. Therefore, at my clinic we advise that slimming diets which recommend high quantities of protein are to be avoided.

Of the 20 amino acids that proteins are made up of, we can manufacture many in our own bodies. However, eight have to be provided in the diet; these are therefore known as *essential* amino acids. Animal proteins supply all the essential amino acids, but vegetarians who eat a varied diet will also easily fulfil their protein requirements. Some women I work with who are vegetarian come to me thinking that if they want to get pregnant they need to start eating chicken or meat. This isn't true, and in fact it is now thought that one of the advantages of a good vegetarian diet is that it contains adequate but not excessive protein.

Vegetarians should aim to obtain protein from:

- Nuts such as almonds, Brazil nuts, cashews and peanut butter
- Seeds such as sesame, sunflower and pumpkin
- Pulses such as chickpeas (including hummus), lentils and beans (including baked beans)
- Dairy products, particularly low-fat ones such as yoghurt and cottage cheese
- Free-range organic eggs
- Fruits and vegetables – all fruits and vegetables contain varying amounts of protein – frozen peas and cooked spinach are particularly high
- Limit soya products to three portions a week – there has been some evidence that too much soya may act as a contraceptive and affect fertility.

The most important thing to remember is to eat a variety of these foods to get a balance of all the amino acids.

Protein Content of Different Foods

1 portion bolognese sauce	28g
1 portion roast chicken breast	27g
1 cup cottage cheese	26g
1 small tin tuna or poached cod fillet	24g
100g tofu	23g
1 cup of porridge oats (raw as in muesli)	16g
1 cup split peas (as in soups and casseroles)	16g
1 cup kidney beans	15g
8 oz low-fat, plain yoghurt	13g

1 cup baked beans	12g
1 oz (142) pumpkin seeds	9g
3 tbs lentils	9g
1 cup semi-skimmed milk	8g
1 cup frozen peas	8g
1 oz cheddar cheese	7g
1 cup of porridge oats (cooked)	7g
1 cup wholewheat spaghetti	7g
1 medium-sized egg	6g
23 dry-roasted, salt-free peanuts	6g
1 cup tinned sweetcorn	5g
1 baked potato	5g
1 cup cooked brown rice	5g
1oz sunflower seeds	5g
1 cup cooked spinach	5g
7 walnut halves	4g
1 tbs peanut butter	4g
1 cup mashed potato with milk	4g
1 small cup seedless raisins	4g
12 almonds	3g
1 oz pine nuts	3g
1 cup okra	3g
1 slice wholemeal bread	3g
1 tbs hummus	2g
3 Brazil nuts	2g
1 plain granola bar	2g
1 cup tinned tomatoes	2g

Protein Meals

Breakfast

Smoothie with seeds, nuts, oats, fruit and semi-skimmed milk	20g
8 oz yoghurt with mixed seeds	19g
Smoothie with seeds, nuts, oats, fruit and oat/rice milk	13g
2 slices wholemeal toast with peanut butter	10g
1 boiled egg, 1 slice wholemeal toast and a glass of orange juice	10g

Lunch

Baked potato with baked beans and cheddar cheese	24g
Baked potato with cottage cheese and salad	20g
Wholegrain (wheat or rye) sandwich with ½ tin tuna or chicken and salad	18g
Soups containing pulses such as Fresh & Wild's Minted Green Pea	17g

Dinner

Chicken fillet with broccoli and mashed potato	40g
Spaghetti (brown) Bolognaise	35g
Salmon fillet with rice and frozen peas	35g

2 nut burgers (nuts, beans, oatmeal and an egg), sweetcorn and spinach	32g
Vegetable casserole with beans and quinoa and rice	25g

Snacks

Banana and mango smoothie with 250ml semi-skimmed milk	10g
1 tbs hummus and 2 oatcakes	5g
1 tbs nuts and seeds	5g
Granola bar	2g
1 small banana	1g

Carbohydrates

Carbohydrates get a bad press, but they are vitally important for energy. Again, it's about the *type* of carbohydrates you eat, and the balance of carbs within your diet. Complex carbohydrates, which use energy over a period of time during digestion, are more beneficial than simple carbohydrates such as refined sugar, which give you a quick burst, elevate insulin levels and cause fluctuations in the blood sugar level that can affect the functioning of other body systems, including hormone production and mood. In order to balance blood sugar levels, and avoid the see-saw effect of high levels of blood sugar that stimulate excessive insulin secretion (which can have a role to play in PCOS – see page 263), you need to eat complex carbohydrates with protein. This combination is greatly beneficial in balancing blood sugar levels.

Simple carbohydrates like refined sugar products, bread, etc. are all too easy to enjoy, but they also produce alcohols that are toxic to the body. Highly refined foods are also acid-producers. Opt for carbohydrates such as potatoes (which are also a good alkaline food), oats, and breads and pasta made from wholewheat rather than refined flour.

The secret to your carbohydrate intake is to eat none in the late evening. Eat your daily intake at breakfast and lunchtime, but reduce your intake after that. Eating carbohydrates at night means they stay longer in the system, allowing more time for the production of alcohols, which in turn need detoxing and elimination from the body, wasting valuable nutritional resources better used for achieving pregnancy.

Low carbs or no carbs can make you feel very depressed, and also reduce your serotonin levels. Serotonin is very important for the womb lining.

Fats

While you only need a small proportion of fat in the diet, this is a good energy source and in some cases provides essential fatty acids (EFAs). These fatty acids, which are (as their name tells us) essential to the body, cannot be manufactured and must come from the diet. While most people are familiar with omega-3 and omega-6 fatty acids, they are not always so clear on what these are, how they work, in what ratio they should appear in the diet, and where they are available from in the diet.

Omega-3 and omega-6 fatty acids are truly essential, particularly for brain development and function, but can't be manufactured by the body so must be provided by the diet. From these EFAs, the body can then make the complex, highly unsaturated fatty acids (HUFAs). However, this process is easily inhibited, especially by a high intake of processed foods, lack of vitamin and mineral co-factors, or prolonged stress – in short, by the main features of the typical Western diet and lifestyle.

- Do you have dry hair?
- Dry skin?
- Cracked nails?
- Poor memory?
- Poor co-ordination?
- Clumsiness?
- Frequent infections?
- Fatigue?
- Allergies or food intolerances?
- PMS and breast tenderness?
- Rough goose bumps on your arms?

You're not getting enough of the right kind of fats in your diet!

Omega-3 and omega-6 are not just good fats – they're essential, and they are also helpful in regulating hormonal function and reducing immunological disturbances, while the EFAs in flaxseed oil are thought to help reduce swelling and inflammation. EFAs are also essential for healthy sperm production and function.

Monounsaturated and polyunsaturated fats are fine in moderate quantities; the ones to avoid are saturated, hydrogenated or 'trans' fats, especially as they promote the formation of free radicals (see below). The antioxidant vitamins A, C and E and the mineral selenium can eliminate free radicals, but your body needs these substances to enhance fertility, so you should try to avoid using up your reserves on combating free radicals in the body.

DHA

I have been talking about DHA being as important as folic acid for years, not least because 8 out of 10 women are deficient in this essential fatty acid. I encourage all women to take it prior to conceiving, as it takes at least three months to be incorporated into the system. It is very much needed in early pregnancy, as it is for brain and eye development in the foetus from 28 weeks.

DHA is also needed for good hormone production, and for this reason I get all of my women clients on four capsules of DHA a day when going through an IVF cycle. It's important for men, too, because sperm contains high concentrations of DHA. Several studies have shown a correlation between the ability of sperm to fertilize eggs and sperm's DHA content, with a deficiency in this causing problems. DHA in men is highly concentrated in the testicles.

Water

Water is essential to life, and an important part of nutrition. I think the message is finally getting across about how important adequate hydration of the body – which is 70 per cent water – is for good health. Although we get quite a lot of liquid from our foods, and from beverages like tea and coffee, the latter two can also have a dehydrating effect. Water should also be a part of everyone's daily liquid intake.

Water is important for a variety of reasons. It is necessary to the body's circulation systems, both of blood and lymph. A good liquid intake, and well-hydrated body, help to create a well-functioning blood circulation, in which nutrients and hormones are transported, and maintain blood pressure so the kidneys work well. Adequate hydration is also necessary for the production of both cervical mucus in the female and prostate fluid in the male (prostate fluid provides the essential medium of semen, in which sperm swim and survive).

Although tap water is safe to drink, it is not the best choice as it very often contains added fluoride; if fluoride levels are high, this can affect your thyroid and consequently your fertility. Chlorine can also be harmful. If you fill a jug of tap water and leave it to stand, most of the chlorine will evaporate off. If you filter your water, using a carbonated filter, you will improve its quality and taste further. You may also consider installing a water-filtration system (invest in one that goes under the sink). At the very least, using a water filter jug will improve the water you drink.

Bottled water varies. Some mineral waters can be very high in sodium, while others can be beneficial because they include magnesium and calcium. But buying bottled water is expensive; it's better to make sure you drink enough rather than be restricted by cost.

Increasing the amount you drink needs to be done progressively over a period of time. You can't re-hydrate your body by going from a poor intake to high intake overnight. As with a dried-out pot plant, a large quantity of water can't be absorbed all at once. But once the plant's soil is re-hydrated, it can hold more water than before. So it is with your body's cells. The recommended amount is 2 litres a day per 50 kilos in body weight.

When water is in short supply, the body will ensure that the organs vital for life receive what they need, before the reproductive system, which is of relatively low priority. To ensure that the reproductive system gets what it needs in terms of hydration, your overall daily consumption has to be adequate. Think of the way a plum becomes a prune through dehydration: you want your body cells to be plums, not prunes! This is key when it comes to the ovaries and womb. Adequate hydration means plump follicles and a strong blood supply to the womb lining, ensuring the lining is well able to nurture and nourish a fertilized egg. The same goes for sperm health and motility: adequate hydration helps prevent clumping of the sperm, and ensures that the semen provides a good environment for movement.

Vitamins and Minerals

Ideally these should come from your diet but, given what we know not just about what we eat but also our eating habits and their effect on the digestive system, I do recommend a good multi-vitamin and -mineral as well as EFA supplement for couples when they are trying to get pregnant, or experiencing problems getting pregnant. A good diet that includes a substantial range of strongly alkaline foods will ensure a good vitamin intake, but it is worth bearing in mind that the water-soluble vitamins B and C need to be replenished daily.

The B vitamins, which cannot be stored in the body, are many and various, and have a major role to play. Folic acid, for example, is recommended as a supplement for all women planning a pregnancy, and during the first three months because it helps avoid the risk of spina bifida, a neural-tube defect that can occur shortly after conception.

Vitamin C is important for ovarian health and collagen, and the absorption of dietary iron. Vitamin E limits oxidative damage in the body (see 'Free Radicals', page 131). While the RDA (Recommended Daily Allowance) of 60mg isn't, in my view, adequate for couples who want to conceive, it's important that women don't take more than a gram (1,000mg) a day because of its anti-histamine effect. This effect can dry up mucus secretions, which makes cervical mucus less prolific – and at ovulation when it's necessary to transport and protect sperm, this is essential.

Vitamin B_1, or thiamine, is essential for ovulation and implantation. Vitamin B_5 is necessary for the clearance of excess oestrogen and progesterone. If these two hormones accumulate in the liver, they can inhibit the release of GNRH, which is necessary for the stimulation of FSH (follicle-stimulating hormone) and LH (luteinizing hormone). B_5 is also necessary for maintaining a balance between oestrogen and progesterone.

Vitamin B_{12} is essential for the cell DNA. A diet low in this B vitamin can slow down the ripening of the egg prior to ovulation.

Zinc, magnesium and vitamin A are important for egg production, and for sperm production. The antioxidant vitamins A, C and E, plus selenium and Co-enzyme Q10, are necessary for the elimination of free radicals, which occur along with oxidization and can damage the body's cells. Co-enzyme Q10 is also beneficial for improving blood flow to the ovaries, and helps sperm, which is why I include it in my recommendations.

Research has shown that for couples wanting to conceive, dietary improvements might not be enough immediately; a good vitamin and mineral supplement is necessary, too. Numerous pieces of research suggest that a couple's chances of conception, and carrying a baby to term, are increased by taking a vitamin and mineral supplement.

I believe in the body's ability to restore balance and to heal. For so many of the couples I see, the balance has gone and some are taking mega-doses of supplements. Very often, looking at their questionnaires and their digestive profile, they are not absorbing the vitamins and minerals they are taking and not making some of the lifestyle changes necessary. Many women think that if they take enough supplements, all will be well. This is not true; you have to put some groundwork in. By making improvements in your diet and lifestyle, the body will rebalance itself.

How Do I Know If I Have a Vitamin Deficiency?

A question I frequently get asked is 'How do I know if I am deficient in a certain vitamin or mineral?' This is a hard one to answer; the only way to find out for sure is to have a blood test, which is very expensive. Nor do I do hair mineral analyses anymore. I believe it causes far too much stress in my clients, and tend instead to look at a couple's overall lifestyle when trying to determine whether they're getting enough of the important nutrients in their diet. I also look at vitamin and mineral profiles. I honestly believe that when you give your system a rest, replenish it with good foods and make lifestyle changes, it restores itself and regains balance.

Free Radicals
Free radicals are a normal by-product of cell chemistry, and occur when a molecule in a body cell isn't paired, or balanced, by another – these 'loose molecules' have to scavenge to find another molecule to pair with. It's this scavenging process that can cause damage to other body cells, and in doing so create a chain-reaction of free radicals.

Some free radicals arise in the body during metabolism; this is normal. And sometimes the body's immune system's cells deliberately create free radicals to neutralize viruses and bacteria. But free radicals are also produced by:

- Smoking
- Processed foods, particularly foods high in artificial additives
- Fast foods
- Alcohol
- Recreational drugs
- Foods that contain high amounts of poor-quality fats and oils, particularly processed meats, margarines, biscuits and pastries, and take-aways.
- Fried, barbecued and burnt foods
- Exposure to environmental pollution such as traffic fumes.

Normally the body can handle free radicals, but if antioxidants (vitamins A, C and E, in particular) are unavailable, or if the free-radical production becomes excessive, damage can occur. The Government recommendation of 'five-a-day' – five portions of vegetables and/or fruits a day – is one way of ensuring an adequate intake of antioxidants. Free radicals can go on to disrupt the DNA of cells in the body, and are implicated in many diseases such as cancer and heart disease.

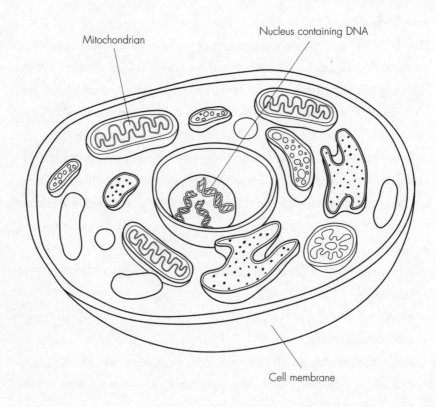

Mitochondrian

Nucleus containing DNA

Cell membrane

In small quantities, and balanced out by a nutritious diet that contains adequate antioxidants, free radicals cause little harm – they are just part of the body's metabolic process – but for many of us, exposed to daily toxins and with an inadequate diet, they become a problem. Free radical damage is also accumulative, and something that increases as we age – easy to see through the effect on our skin, for example!

When immune cells are damaged by free radicals they no longer recognize invading alien cells, and this can lead to auto-immune diseases, where the body destroys its own tissues. When it comes to fertility, reducing free radical damage is important. Taking vitamin and mineral supplements can help, as well as improving your intake through the foods you eat every day.

There is a lot of evidence now to show that free radical damage can affect the DNA of the sperm and the eggs. Free radical damage in the body is caused by environmental factors, such as cigarettes, alcohol and barbecued foods, and the chemical pollutants in everyday life. These can be improved upon by detoxing – see page 141.

The Role of Homocysteine

Homocysteine is an amino acid, a building block of protein, produced by the body and normally changed into other amino acids that the body can use. Vitamin B is necessary for this natural process to occur; without vitamin B there may not be enough enzymes for this to happen. A raised homocysteine level can be a problem, as it irritates blood vessels, roughening them and allowing plaque to accumulate, which can lead to blockages in the arteries (atherosclerosis). High homocysteine levels in the blood can also cause cholesterol to change to a form that is more damaging to arteries (called oxidized low-density lipoprotein).

In addition, high homocysteine levels can make blood clot more easily than it should, increasing the risk of blood-vessel blockages. This can be a problem when you are trying to conceive, and particularly at implantation and when the placenta starts to develop. When it comes to fertility, high levels of homocysteine have been linked to early miscarriage, and to low levels of oestrogen and progesterone.

Most people with a high homocysteine level have a low dietary intake of folate (also called folic acid), vitamin B_6 or vitamin B_{12}. Replacing these vitamins in a supplement helps the homocysteine level return to normal. Other possible causes of an abnormally high homocysteine level include low thyroid hormone levels, kidney disease, psoriasis, and some medications or inherited deficiencies in the enzymes used to process homocysteine in the body.

A healthy homocysteine level is less than 12 mmol per litre (L). A level of greater than 12 mmol per L is considered high. However, I wouldn't want any of you, reading this, to go running off to your GP to be tested – just take steps to ensure you are getting an adequate level of B vitamins, and aren't depleting yourself by drinking too much alcohol.

- Eating more fruits and vegetables (especially leafy green vegetables) can help lower your homocysteine level.
- Good sources of dietary folate include many breakfast cereals, lentils, chickpeas, asparagus, spinach and most beans.
- If this isn't enough to lower your homocysteine level, you will also need to take specific vitamins. You may need to take a fairly large amount of folate (about 1mg per day). Additional vitamin B_6 and vitamin B_{12} will also help the body process homocysteine. In addition to vitamin B, selenium is important, as is magnesium.
- There is much research now to show that free radical damage affects the developing embryo. It is really important when you do get pregnant to take 1g (1,000 mg) of vitamin C and 400iu of vitamin E daily.

Fertility and Your Weight

If you are a woman who is heavily overweight, or seriously underweight, you will find it harder to conceive. In addition, you probably won't be accepted on an IVF programme if you are extremely over- or underweight, so addressing this straight away is essential.

Fat is the most changeable, labile tissue in the body. It is the first tissue that recognizes and responds to changes in the environment such as your food intake and physical activity levels. The brain responds to how fat or thin you are by turning off your menstrual cycle. Oestrogen deposited in body fat can convert to androgens, which are male hormones. Fat of the breast and abdomen all make oestrogen, and oestrogen is made in the fatty marrow of the long bones. If there is too much oestrogen in your body, your hormone balance will be adversely affected.

We help our overweight clients to lose weight, because we explain to them that losing 10 per cent of their body weight will help their chances of conceiving considerably. Easier said than done, I know, especially if you suffer from PCOS (see page 263).

People sometimes ask me why weight matters, if a woman is healthy, but excess weight affects hormone production, which we know is critical to a woman's ability to ovulate and get pregnant. Fat cells constantly release oestrogen, which will inhibit FSH (follicle-stimulating hormone) production by the pituitary gland, preventing ovulation.

Equally, a seriously underweight woman probably won't ovulate regularly, as her body goes into 'survival mode' and the diminished hormones also mean that if she does ovulate, she won't necessarily produce adequate hormones to allow the pregnancy to continue. Too few fat cells mean too little oestrogen, which can also affect cervical mucus secretion. You only need to be 10 per cent at odds with the optimum weight for your height for your hormone balance to be affected.

For some women this may not matter at all; for others it makes a profound difference.

Some of the women who are underweight do have past issues with anorexia and bulimia; they generally also overestimate what they are eating in a day. Very often they read labels and are still conscious of products that contain fat, so very often go for low-fat products, which are full of chemicals that are bad for you. Many women also exercise too much, finding room for exercise in their lifestyles rather than good, healthy foods.

Nutritious Foods for Gaining Weight in Preparation for Pregnancy

The key is to eat both calorie- *and* nutrient-rich foods, not to suddenly start eating more junk foods with empty calories.

- Olive oil – buy cold-pressed, organic unrefined and have it with vegetables and bread and use plenty in cooking. Mix with walnut oil for salads, and sesame oil for stir-fries
- Avocados
- All plain nuts
- Seeds
- Coconut milk – can be used in Indian and Thai curries, and is also delicious in smoothies
- Dried fruit – make good snacks and are delicious soaked, poached and pureed
- Oily fish like salmon (organic or wild), mackerel, herrings, sardines
- Mayonnaise – add garlic and fresh herbs and use as a dip with home-made potato crisps roasted in olive oil
- Hummus (not low fat)
- Sun-dried tomatoes and pesto

- Full-fat natural organic yoghurt
- Bananas
- Home-made carrot, banana or date and walnut cake

Case History: Gemma

Gemma was 30 and had been trying for a baby for two years. She had a past history of anorexia. Her BMI was 19 (that is, very low – the optimal Body Mass Index is between 20 and 25; see below). She worked as a secretary. Over the years she had had a lot of therapy around issues in the past with her mother, but felt she had dealt with them and that these issues were behind her.

Gemma worked hard and went to the gym six times a week: in her lunchtime, during the working week, and at the weekend. She did not eat before going to the gym, and would race back to the office and have a quick sandwich instead. Her diet consisted of low-fat foods, yoghurts, lots of fizzy drinks, few carbohydrates. She was faddy about eating meat.

I spent time with Gemma, finding out about the foods that she did like, and making a list of them. I explained about the impact of the low-fat foods she was eating on her fertility, and advised her to switch to 'real' foods, increase her intake of carbohydrates (baked potatoes and wholemeal breads), cut out the fizzy drinks, cut down on visits to the gym, and eat lunch prior to exercising. I also advised her to start adding good fats to her diet – not cakes or sweets but avocados, olive oil, mayonnaise, and full-fat yoghurts and milk.

BODY MASS INDEX TABLE

	Normal						Overweight					Obese					
BMI	**19**	**20**	**21**	**22**	**23**	**24**	**25**	**26**	**27**	**28**	**29**	**30**	**31**	**32**	**33**	**34**	**35**
58	91	96	100	105	110	115	119	124	129	134	138	143	148	153	158	162	167
59	94	99	104	109	114	119	124	128	133	138	143	148	153	158	163	168	173
60	97	102	107	112	118	123	128	133	138	143	148	153	158	163	168	174	179
61	100	106	111	116	122	127	132	137	143	148	153	158	164	169	174	180	185
62	104	109	115	120	126	131	136	142	147	153	158	164	169	175	180	186	191
63	107	113	118	124	130	135	141	146	152	158	163	169	175	180	186	191	197
64	110	116	122	128	134	140	145	151	157	163	169	174	180	186	192	197	204
65	114	120	126	132	138	144	150	156	162	168	174	180	186	192	198	204	210
66	118	124	130	136	142	148	155	161	167	173	179	186	192	198	204	210	216
67	121	127	134	140	146	153	159	166	172	178	185	191	198	204	211	217	223
68	125	131	138	144	151	158	164	171	177	184	190	197	203	210	216	223	230
69	128	135	142	149	155	162	169	176	182	189	196	203	209	216	223	230	236
70	132	139	146	153	160	167	174	181	188	195	202	209	216	222	229	236	243
71	136	143	150	157	165	172	179	186	193	200	208	215	222	229	236	243	250
72	140	147	154	162	169	177	184	191	199	206	213	221	228	235	242	250	258
73	144	151	159	166	174	182	189	197	204	212	219	227	235	242	250	257	265
74	148	155	163	171	179	186	194	202	210	218	225	233	241	249	256	264	272
75	152	160	168	176	184	192	200	208	216	224	232	240	248	256	264	272	279
76	156	164	172	180	189	197	205	213	221	230	238	246	254	263	271	279	287

Height (inches) (left axis label)

Body weight (pounds)

				Extreme obesity														
36	37	38	39	40	41	42	43	44	45	46	47	48	49	50	51	52	53	54
172	177	181	186	191	196	201	205	210	215	220	224	229	234	239	244	248	253	258
178	183	188	193	198	203	208	212	217	222	227	232	237	242	247	252	257	262	267
184	189	194	199	204	209	215	220	225	230	235	240	245	250	255	261	266	271	276
190	195	201	206	211	217	222	227	232	238	243	248	254	259	264	269	275	280	285
196	202	207	213	218	224	229	235	240	246	251	256	262	267	273	278	284	289	295
203	208	214	220	225	231	237	242	248	254	259	265	270	278	282	287	293	299	304
209	215	221	227	232	238	244	250	256	262	267	273	279	285	291	296	302	308	314
216	222	228	234	240	246	252	258	264	270	276	282	288	294	300	306	312	318	324
223	229	235	241	247	253	260	266	272	278	284	291	297	303	309	315	322	328	334
230	236	242	249	255	261	268	274	280	287	293	299	306	312	319	325	331	338	344
236	243	249	256	262	269	276	282	289	295	302	308	315	322	328	335	341	348	354
243	250	257	263	270	277	284	291	297	304	311	318	324	331	338	345	351	358	365
250	257	264	271	278	285	292	299	306	313	320	327	334	341	348	355	362	369	376
257	265	272	279	286	293	301	308	315	322	329	338	343	351	358	365	372	379	386
265	272	279	287	294	302	309	316	324	331	338	346	353	361	368	375	383	390	397
272	280	288	295	302	310	318	325	333	340	348	355	363	371	378	386	393	401	408
280	287	295	303	311	319	326	334	342	350	358	365	373	381	389	396	404	412	420
287	295	303	311	319	327	335	343	351	359	367	375	383	391	399	407	415	423	431
295	304	312	320	328	336	344	353	361	369	377	385	394	402	410	418	426	435	443

Source: Adapted from *Clinical Guidelines on the Identification, Evaluation, and Treatment of Overweight and Obesity in Adults: The Evidence Report.*

BMI

To find out if you are the right weight for your height, you need to work out your BMI (Body Mass Index). Divide your weight (in kilograms) by your height (in metres) squared. A BMI of less than 18.5 means you are underweight, while a BMI of over 25 means you are overweight.

If you are overweight, don't be tempted to crash diet – you need a sustained, nutritionally sound weight-loss programme. Equally, if you are underweight it's worth looking at why, and choosing a balanced, high-calorie diet to help you gain weight healthily. In either case, consulting a nutritionist is advisable.

Most women I know do have emotional relationships with food. So it is not just about losing weight, but for some of you, it is getting to the bottom of what that relationship is.

We do a weight-loss control programme under the supervision of a nutritionist or dietician. The guidelines in this chapter form the basis for this. We also recommend you keep a food diary, as many people with weight problems do tend to underestimate the amount they eat.

Useful Tips

- It takes the brain 15 minutes to recognize the feeling of fullness.
- Do not use your body as a dustbin, eating up all the leftovers: Save them for lunch or supper.
- Always eat breakfast.
- Try not to add salt to your food (salt encourages water retention).
- Be careful about portion control.
- If you have big plates, start using smaller ones.
- Cut down on foods with fat such as sausages, ham and bacon.
- Wean yourself off the need for something sweet after dinner.

- Exercise is a crucial part of any weight loss programme (see page 183).
- Avoid the use of low-fat products as they contain chemicals and artificial sweeteners. You are far better with a natural product – a small amount of butter or cream is far better for you.

Aim to lose 2 lb a week and do not punish yourself if you have a few slip-ups along the way.

A Detox Programme

Every day our bodies absorb chemicals from the foods we eat, the air we breathe and the products we use. For most of us, our day-to-day environment provides a lot of pollutants with which the body has to contend, from alcohol and cigarette smoke to car exhaust, pesticides and preservatives.

Generally, if the body is well rested, well exercised and well functioning, these pollutants are counterbalanced and can be dealt with quite efficiently. However, for most of us the everyday toxic load isn't well dealt with and the effects of this can build up until they produce anything from a minor allergy to a full-blown illness. I believe that regular detoxing once or twice a year is key to maintaining good health, and never is it more important – for both partners – than if you are trying to conceive, whether naturally or through assisted conception.

What a detox will do for you is re-establish hormonal balance, because production of all our hormones starts with a good digestive system. This is very, very important.

If you answered yes to any of the questions on page 99, then it is likely that your digestive system is not functioning to its best capacity, and a detox will help.

The detoxification process – which occurs through all the excretory organs, the skin, lungs and lymphatic system as well as the bowels and kidneys – helps all the body systems work more effectively. This means that digestion is improved, along with hormonal balance. The lymph system, sleep, exercise, meditation and breathing all have an effect on our fertility and can't be separated.

How a Detox Works

For the body to eliminate the waste products of metabolism efficiently, the excretory organs have to be working well. The organs of excretion are the liver, the skin, the lungs, the kidneys and the intestines. If one or more of these organs are compromised in some way, then greater pressure is landed on the others to ensure that effective excretion of metabolic and environmental toxins occurs. If the detoxification organs become overwhelmed, the emphasis is on keeping the blood clear, so toxins get deposited in the body. So, for a full detoxification and to restore balance in the body, these toxins need to be drawn back from the cells of the body into the blood and to the organs of detoxification for excretion.

The Colon

The colon is the organ of elimination for metabolic refuse, and is where a large percentage of the immune cells are made. Colon-cleansing is a very important part of any detox. A sluggish digestive system, where waste products remain in transit for an extended length of time, means that the opportunity for toxicity is increased. As the colon is also the organ of reabsorption, two things can happen: toxins can be generated (alcohol from the fermentation of fruit and vegetable waste, for example) which are then reabsorbed if waste products spend too long in transit, and the waste – or faeces – can become very dry and difficult to pass. Constipation and impacted faeces can become a problem for many, not least because they restrict the muscular contractions of the bowel, and women in particular can be doubly affected as the smooth muscle of the bowel is also affected by the hormone progesterone.

The knock-on effect of an ill-functioning colon is on the liver. The greater the length of time food waste spends in transit, the greater the opportunity for the production of additional toxins and metabolic wastes that are reabsorbed into the bloodstream, requiring detoxification in the liver. The single most common cause of colon inefficacy is a poor diet.

The Liver

The liver is the most potent chemical detoxifier in the body, so during a detox it's important to support your liver. The health of the liver is the primary goal in this diet, and we have focused on this as well as on regaining and maintaining hormonal balance.

The Kidneys

The kidneys excrete urine, and are also responsible for the selective reabsorption of liquid, and to maintain the body's electrolyte balance. A healthy person should excrete between 3 and 4 pints (1 and 1½ litres) of urine a day, which should be of a clear, light amber colour if hydration is adequate.

The Skin

The skin is a very effective detoxification organ. We excrete a lot of metabolic waste through our skin, including urea (from which urine is made) in our perspiration. The skin's excretory potential can be increased through daily body brushing – see page 148.

In Traditional Chinese Medicine, the health of the skin is linked to the colon and lungs. One way to enhance the function of the skin is to bathe in a bath to which Epsom salts have been added. Immersing the body in a salt saturated solution encourages the body to excrete fluid via the skin, reducing puffiness. Puffiness may be the result of a high-salt diet, making the body cells retain fluid to ensure that the balance of salts in the body is kept stable. Cut down your intake of salt – we tend to eat more than is good for us, anyway – the body cells will retain less fluid, and you will have less puffiness.

The Lymphatic System

Lymph is a clear fluid that contains numerous proteins, but most importantly lymphocytes, which form part of the body's immune system. The effectiveness of the lymphatic system in detoxification should not be underestimated. Just as with the blood system, the lymphatic system has its own circulation and is designed to assist in the removal of waste products from the cells of the body. Unlike the circulation of the blood, however, there is no pump (the heart); instead the lymphatic system has to rely on muscular body movement to assist circulation. Lymph vessels have valves to prevent back-flow, but rely on the contraction of the surrounding muscles to squeeze lymph along its way.

Over 20 per cent of white blood corpuscles are lymphocytes, which consist of B lymphocytes, which produce antibodies, and T lymphocytes, which attack and destroy antigens. Lymph also provides a medium with which to absorb and transport toxins and cell waste in the body to the lymph nodes for cleansing. A sluggish lymphatic system means that this system of waste disposal is compromised, and the body suffers from a build-up of stagnant lymph.

The lymphatic system also plays a key role in the circulation of hormones. If it is not functioning well, this can delay the circulation of fertility hormones. Lymphatic stasis, (which means there is little movement), can also affect the feedback-system of fertility hormones, and as a woman's fertility cycle relies on this feedback system working effectively, problems can arise. For example, it is the peak oestrogen level that stimulates the production of luteinizing hormone (LH), which in turn stimulates the release of an egg (ovulation).

Lymphatic fluid filters many substances from the body, but it is a system that can become very sluggish and ineffectual, not least because of our sedentary lifestyles and high-sodium diets. One way of enhancing the effectiveness of the lymphatic system during a detox is through Manual Lymphatic Drainage. This is an extremely gentle but effective way of supporting and stimulating the system to work better. It is also of value during pregnancy and post-natally, but in relation to pre-conception, MLD helps with the following:

- balancing hormones and regulating a woman's periods
- boosting the performance of the immune system
- detoxifying
- relieving fluid congestion
- helping with symptoms of PMS
- deeply relaxing and helpful for stress relief
- aiding digestion and helping with disorders such as IBS (Irritable Bowel Syndrome)
- improving sleep quality

Manual Lymphatic Drainage Massage

By its name, it may sound like Manual Lymphatic Drainage (MLD) means you are about to have the whole of your lymphatic system drained away, but it is actually a very gentle form of massage aimed at moving the lymph just under the skin. I use this treatment as part of any recommended nutrition and detox plans, to help prepare for conception, for IVF treatment, in between IVF treatments and after a miscarriage.

MLD was developed by the Danish physiotherapist Dr Emil Vodder in the 1930s, and involves light, rhythmical massage that aids the body in collecting and moving lymphatic fluid. This plays a key role in delivering nutrients and antibodies to where they are needed, and removing debris such as toxins, cell waste and dead particles for cleansing. MLD also works on the nervous system, lowering blood pressure, reducing stress and improving sleep patterns.

Because we recognize that our clients have busy lives, we have tried to create a detox programme that will not cause drastic side-effects. There is **no** fasting, no skipping meals, replacing meals or eating only one or two different foods. You will eat three small, healthy meals as well as snacks and even puddings. We have included fish, chicken, eggs and yoghurt, as clients preparing for pregnancy have more specific needs for protein, iron, zinc and vitamin B_{12}.

An effective detox should be approached gradually: cutting out coffee one week, alcohol the next week and sugar the next, so that when you do the full 48-hour detox the impact is not so dramatic in terms of how you feel.

The detox programme excludes all direct sources of toxins as well as foods such as wheat and dairy for a short period of time, as these can have an irritating effect on the lining of the gastro-intestinal tract. Animal-derived foods are reduced significantly, and fruit and vegetable intake is increased, in order to help cleanse the bowel of toxins, which is important as these bowel toxins can be reabsorbed back into the blood, after which they will pass on to the liver for detoxification. The high fibre intake also encourages the body to excrete any toxins that are already present. A low-fibre diet is associated with an overgrowth of toxin-producing bacteria and a lower level of healthy gastro-intestinal bacteria.

Saturated animal fats (full-fat dairy, fatty meats, creamy cheeses, etc.) are removed from this diet because they encourage the growth of bacteria in the intestine that produce an enzyme which converts oestrogen into a form that can be reabsorbed from the bowel, again preventing efficient clearance. They also contain substances which encourage inflammation. However, 'good' fats such as those found in many nuts and seeds, and fish, are encouraged.

Withdrawal

It is possible that you may experience withdrawal headaches in the first few days; however this usually passes as your body adapts to not having, for example, caffeine, sugar or alcohol. Taking vitamin C and drinking at least 2 litres of water during this period will help to minimize these symptoms.

Do not attempt a detox if you suspect you may be pregnant. If you are on any medications, don't come off them. If you have diabetes or any other medical condition, do check with your GP before you start a detox.

Certain foods are particularly beneficial in helping to improve the detoxification abilities of the liver, such as garlic, onions, members of the brassica family (broccoli, cabbage and Brussels sprouts), asparagus and avocados. Beans, pulses, onions and garlic contain *methionine*, which assists *methylation*, the chemical process by which the liver breaks down oestrogen.

The liver can be further supported by taking a herbal supplement including silymarin (milk thistle), which is possibly the most potent liver-protector known. Clinical trials have documented the efficacy of silymarin for a variety of liver disorders, and it helps to protect the liver in people undertaking long-term drug programmes, without interfering with the clinical efficacy of their medication.

The liver also needs a plentiful supply of vitamins to aid the detoxification process, so a good-quality prenatal multi-vitamin and -mineral supplement is recommended.

Finally, a supplement of the beneficial bacteria *Lactobacillus acidophilus* is recommended, to help improve the health of the gastro-intestinal tract and reduce possible bowel toxicity.

After you complete the detox programme it's a good idea to continue with a maintenance pre-conceptual health programme. You can adapt this for yourself from the dietary guidelines you will receive at a pre-conceptual consultation.

Extra Help

- Manual lymphatic drainage massage (MLD) is an excellent complementary treatment to the liver detox (see page 145).
- Try skin-brushing, which aids lymphatic drainage. Take a soft, natural-bristle, dry brush and brush your skin (also dry) in long, sweeping strokes in the direction of your heart: from your fingertips to under your arms in long smooth strokes, then from your toes round to the back of your knees, and from your knees to your groin. Gently brush your abdomen in a circular motion from the lower right up and round to the lower left. Brush your chest and shoulders towards your collarbones. You are brushing towards areas which contain lymph nodes, aiding the passage of lymphatic fluid that carries off toxins, and stimulating blood flow.
- Have a sauna or a steam, as this will help to 'sweat' out toxins through the skin. Saunas encourage sweating (but be sure to rehydrate afterwards with lots of filtered water), which is a good way of helping the skin excrete toxins more effectively. But please note: this is not to be done if you might be pregnant.

- Use detoxifying essential oils in your bath: Add 5 drops of lemon, lavender and cypress oils to warm water and soak for at least 10 minutes.
- Don't do vigorous exercise during this period, just brisk walking in the fresh air and sunshine will help the detoxification process. The effect of sunlight on the pineal gland enhances a feeling of well-being, and combined with a 20-minute walk helps stimulate lymphatic flow, too. Sunlight on the skin also promotes the production of vitamin D. Although excessive sunbathing is not good for the skin, exposure to sunlight every day is important to our health.
- Try deep breathing techniques (see page 186), yoga and swimming.
- Get plenty of sleep.

Finally, choose a time when you are able to rest a little during the detox process, maybe over a long weekend to begin with, or during a holiday period.

If you are going to have to work while you detox, forward planning is very important. Make a big batch of soup which you can freeze in individual portions to take to work in a flask, prepare salads the night before, have your breakfast ingredients to hand in the morning and keep a ready supply of fruits, nuts, seeds, fruit smoothies and non-dairy milk at work, as well as herbal tea bags, dandelion or barley/dandelion coffee and a big bottle of water.

If you don't manage it, don't worry – keep going, as even a couple of days can have a beneficial effect on liver health and regeneration.

Try to have a relaxing therapeutic treatment during this time – a massage, facial, reflexology or aromatherapy treatment – as this will also help the detoxification process.

Case History: Sarah

Sarah was age 32 when she came to the clinic. Her partner's sperm was average. They had been trying for a baby for four years and were waiting to do IVF, so came in order to prepare. Her cycle was 21 to 30 days and she had no idea of when her fertile time was.

Looking at her questionnaire, I felt that the biggest factors affecting her chances of conceiving were her weight, which was 13 stone (182 lb) – Sarah was 5 foot 10 – her diet and her painkiller intake. Sarah had had a bad riding accident eight years previously and was now on eight painkillers a day on a bad day. She also had no idea that these might be having an effect on her fertility. She hardly ever ate breakfast – and when she did it was sugar puffs, white bread and jam. She drank 20 cups of tea a day, all with sweeteners, plus four cans of diet cola. Her mid-afternoon snacks were mini chocolate rolls. No water, no veg, no fruit. Ready-made evening meals. Little wonder that among her other health problems were constipation and indigestion!

Sarah got up early to go to work, so was worried about having time to eat properly first thing. We helped her to plan ahead at the weekend to prepare for the week ahead, and encourage her to try and get up 20 minutes earlier to fit breakfast in.

The aim for Sarah was to:

1. Lose weight
2. Reduce her painkiller intake
3. Change and improve her diet.

It is dangerous ever to cut everything out, as tempting as it may be. You need to do things gradually.

For her diet, we first got Sarah to eat breakfast – a really important meal of the day. And no more sugar puffs! Instead, porridge, or eggs and wholemeal toast, yoghurt, linseeds, fresh juice, home-made muesli, water and a cup of tea. Sarah reduced her tea-drinking to four cups a day, without sweetener, and stopped drinking diet cola. Instead, she started drinking a litre of water a day.

For lunch: baked potatoes with beans, hummus, rice, salads, pasta, carrots, celery, peppers, avocados and fruit.

Evening meal: lots of steamed vegetables, grilled chicken or fish, omelettes.

We did this for two weeks, then introduced a detox.

To reduce Sarah's painkiller intake, we worked with her GP and started electro-acupuncture on points on her legs and knees on a weekly basis, plus introduced her to using a TENS machine at night, showing her which acupuncture points to use with the pads. Hypnotherapy also helped with pain relief, as well as self-help techniques to manage the pain. After a week Sarah was able to reduce her painkiller intake by two tablets a day, which lessened still further over the next few weeks until she was off them completely.

We built up Sarah's digestive system by introducing probiotics to strengthen her gut. We increased her essential fatty acids and prescribed a multi-vitamin and -mineral.

Sarah gradually began to lose weight, came off the painkillers and, perhaps most importantly, began to understand more about her own fertility. She went on to become pregnant naturally. If this seems like a miracle, it's not. It is common sense and looking at the overall picture.

Detox Diet

This is a sample detox diet to do over a weekend. If you are going to try it for any longer than this, you need to do so under the supervision of a healthcare professional.

There are three groups of food: in the **BOLD** group are the foods that you can eat liberally every day. In the *ITALICS* group are the foods which are restricted to certain days.

The <u>UNDERLINED</u> group foods are to be completely avoided, as these are the ones that cause inflammation and toxicity and are difficult for the liver and digestive system to process.

Foods to be Eaten Liberally

VEGETABLES: as much variety as possible, particularly including:

Alfalfa and other sprouted	**Celery**
vegetables	**Garlic**
Artichokes	**Kale**
Asparagus	**Onions**
Avocado	**Peas**
Beetroot	**Peppers**
Broccoli	**Pumpkin**
Brussels sprouts	**Spinach**
Cabbage	**Sweet potatoes**
Carrots	**Watercress**
Cauliflower	

FRESH HERBS:

Chives	**Parsley**
Coriander – natural detoxifiers	

FRUITS: as much variety as possible, particularly including:

Apples	**Bananas**
Apricots	**Berries – especially blueberries**

Kiwifruit

Lemons – use juice for salad
dressings, and drink the juice
of ½ lemon in hot water
20 minutes before breakfast

Mangoes

Papayas

Peaches

Pears

Pineapple

PULSES:

Beans (cannelloni, flageolet,
butter, kidney, borlotti)

Peas (dried, split yellow,
black-eyed)

Chickpeas (includes hummous)

Lentils (brown, green, red,
yellow)

WHOLE GRAINS/CEREALS:

Amaranth

Barley

Buckwheat

Corn

Millet

Oat bran

Oat germ

Oats

Quinoa

Rye

Wholegrain rice

SEEDS:

Linseeds/flaxseeds (ground
or soaked)

Pumpkin seeds

Sesame seeds (includes tahini)

Sunflower seeds

COLD-PRESSED, UNREFINED NUT AND SEED OILS:

Flax oil

Hazelnut oil

Olive oil

Sesame oil

Walnut oil

WATER:

Filtered, bottled water (naturally sparkling is fine but avoid carbonated
water)

MILKS:

Almond milk (unsweetened)   Oat milk

Rice milk

FRUIT AND VEGETABLE JUICES:

Apple   Carrot

Barley/chicory coffee   Green vegetables

Beetroot   Watermelon (with seeds)

Dandelion 'coffee'   Wheatgrass
  (liver cleanser)

Try beetroot, celery, apple and carrot for a liver detoxifying juice, or carrot,
apple, pear and ginger, or fresh pineapple juice

FRUIT/HERBAL TEAS:

Celestial Seasonings   Fresh ginger tea

Dr Stuart's Botanical Teas   Nettle tea

Essiac tea

Loose herbal teas recommended from Herbs Hands Healing. Check the
ingredients on fruit and herbal teas because they often contain flavourings
and colours.

Foods Restricted to Certain Days

WHITE FISH:

Cod   *Plaice*

Haddock   *Sole*

WHITE MEAT:

Chicken   *Turkey*

Eggs

Live/bio natural yoghurt (low fat if you are trying to lose weight)

Manuka or organic honey

Nuts, particularly almonds, Brazil nuts, walnuts

DRIED FRUITS:

Apricots (try organic without sulphur
  dioxide as a preservative)

Dates

Figs

Prunes

Raisins

Foods to Avoid Completely

Alcohol

Caffeine

Sugar and sweets

REFINED CARBOHYDRATES:

Biscuits

Cakes

Pasta

Pastries

Rice

White bread

Red meat

DAIRY PRODUCTS:

Butter

Cheese

Milk

Wheat

ADDITIVES:

Colours

E numbers

Flavourings

Preservatives

Orange Juice

Trans fats or hydrogenated fats

Packaged and processed foods (including processed meats)

Aspartame and other artificial sweeteners

Salt

Yeast

Organic Foods

Ideally all the food you eat will be relatively free of pesticides and additives. Pesticides are known to be 'hormone-disrupting' chemicals, while organic fruits and vegetables are also believed to contain higher levels of minerals due to the pesticide-free growing conditions and shorter storage time. Pesticides have to be metabolized by the liver and so are an added burden. Many of the antioxidants in plants are made as a defence mechanism by the plant against pests, so removing the pests lowers the levels of these disease-fighting chemicals in plants.

Having said this, many of the foods mentioned are hard to find organically grown and there is also a cost element involved. If nothing else, make sure you choose organic fruits and vegetables, as pesticide use is particularly prevalent in non-organic production. We would also advise that all animal products eaten be organic or at least free-range. They taste better and are less contaminated with hormones, antibiotics and chemical residues.

Liver-friendly Foods

Bitter foods increase bile flow, which helps to remove substances broken down by liver cells:

- Beetroot
- Dandelion ('coffee')
- Chicory
- Radiccio
- Mustard leaves
- Grapefuit
- Lecithin granules (from any good health food shop) can be sprinkled onto food; this helps to break down fats and protects the liver from damage.

Four-Day Detox

(This can also work as the beginning of a weight-loss programme.)
- Days 1, 2 and 4: Eat foods from the **BOLD** group only
- Day 3: Eat foods from both the *ITALICS* and the **BOLD** groups

Sample Menus

Days 1, 2 and 4
Breakfast
- Home-made muesli with different combinations of oat flakes, barley, millet and rye with extra oat germ. Add seeds, such as sunflower, pumpkin and sesame – whole or ground – and ground or soaked lin-seeds and coconut flakes. Add fresh fruit and cinnamon and have with oat or rice milk. Leave to soak for 20 minutes, as this helps to break down the hard husks.
- Stewed fruit compotes, e.g. apples, pears, plums and apricots with added pumpkin seeds

Lunch
- Salads:
- Bean salad – kidney beans, chickpeas, green peas
- Carrot salad – grated carrots, grated apple, thinly sliced red cabbage
- Mixed green salad – rocket, lettuce, watercress, and with millet
- Dressing – olive oil and lemon juice
- Fresh vegetable soup with beans, lentils or chickpeas and a slice of rye bread

Evening Meal

- Steamed vegetables or vegetable stir-fry with mangetout, baby corn, sliced red peppers, carrots, broccoli, onions, onions and garlic, with amaranth, quinoa or buckwheat
- Barley risotto with carrots, onions, garlic, celery and pumpkin seeds

Pudding

- Baked banana

Snacks

- Fruits, fresh fruit smoothies, freshly made fruit and vegetable juices, sunflower and pumpkin seed mix

Day 3
Breakfast

- Muesli: as before, but add yoghurt and nuts
- Fruit compote with yoghurt and mixed seeds

Lunch

(Have fish or chicken for either lunch or dinner but not both.)

- Grilled organic chicken or poached fish with lemon and herbs, salad or steamed vegetables, served with wholegrain rice
- Poached eggs on rye toast

Evening Meal

(Make this predominantly vegetables and very light.)

- Chicken and vegetable stir-fry containing onions, broccoli, red cabbage, carrots, cooked in olive oil and flavoured with garlic, ginger and lemongrass served with amaranth or quinoa
- Sweet potato fish cakes baked in the oven with roasted cherry tomatoes and garlic and a watercress salad

Pudding

* Baked apple and raisins

Snacks

* Fruits, nuts, seeds, dried fruits, smoothies, fresh vegetable juices.

Finally ...

If you experience any pain or discomfort during your detox, please discontinue both the diet and the supplements and contact your GP or nutritionist. If you have been using alcohol, caffeine or cigarettes as stimulants and you have decided to detox, drink a small glass of grapefruit juice with warm water first thing in the morning. This contains a substance called naringenen, which slows down the process between the two stages of detoxification. This can reduce the uncomfortable side-effects – headache, furry tongue, aches and pains – that can sometimes accompany detoxification.

lifestyle factors

Where has all the balance gone?

There are many lifestyle changes that can improve fertility and have huge benefits. Many of the couples I see have to find the balance that has been lacking in their lives. They may be working excessively, drinking too much alcohol or not getting enough sleep or rest – these can have a huge impact on their fertility. I help them to get the balance back into their lives. Everyone's lifestyle is different, and generally couples know where their weaknesses lie and what has to change.

When it comes to balance, however, sometimes the problem can become too much austerity rather than too much excess. I find that some couples who have fertility problems cut out everything, and end up with no life at all, and certainly no social life, for example.

You need to take a step back and look at the areas of your life that could do with improvement. Taking stock, reviewing your lifestyle and re-establishing a balance takes time and thought. One way to kick-start this, which I recommend to couples, is to do a detox (see page 141). A proper detox, giving your system a complete clean-out, involves rest and focusing on the self in all its aspects, and this can't be done without proper commitment.

Work

The most common problem I see among those couples who need to make lifestyle changes has to do with their work and the stress it causes them. So often work demands take priority over all else, and because of our 24-hour society, we never have to switch off from work when laptops, for example, make bringing work home so easy. And it's insidious. Work demands creep up and escalate. The office culture is such that taking time off – even when allowed – can somehow be seen as a sign of weakness. Many, many couples are living to work, rather than working to live, and find it difficult to do otherwise.

The knock-on effect of working 12-hour days is that meals are fast, and often late in the evening, eaten without relaxation or time for proper digestion. This immediately has a detrimental effect on the nutrient content of the meal, which may be compromised anyway if the food is pre-prepared or processed to start with. This may be washed down with regular amounts of alcohol, in an effort to relax, which further compromises your nutritional status. Going to bed late, without any recreation or relaxation, in a stressed state, results in poor sleep. Waking tired, without time for breakfast, and subsisting on instant coffee further depletes energy. It's a vicious circle, and what also gets left out of the equation is the time and inclination for sexual intimacy, without which pregnancy just can't occur, under any circumstances. Time after time I see couples who are basically just not having enough sex to get pregnant.

I am commonly asked by women who are trying to conceive, 'Should I give up work?' My answer is no. If you enjoy what you do, then you should continue to work. Nothing is worse than sitting alone all day, with time on your hands, feeling anxious about conceiving and with little to give your life a sense of purpose or meaning, while you wait to get pregnant. This can be counter-productive in itself. However, do make any changes that will allow you to cut back on your working hours, or reduce the responsibilities that stress you. Discuss with your boss the demands of your working day, and see what can be done to alleviate excessive ones. It's tricky in our work-led lives to see how valuable it might be to create a better work/life balance, but it could be essential in the overall scheme of introducing the sort of balance that may make pregnancy possible.

Admittedly this is tricky for women. They may want to seek other work, but are afraid of changing jobs and then getting pregnant without having accrued any maternity leave – and a new workplace involves new stresses, anyway. Others are afraid that if they let their boss know they are planning a pregnancy, they'll risk being passed over for future promotion. All of this also increases stress in the workplace.

There is no ideal solution, and there are no guarantees, but it is important to take on board the role work plays within your work/life ratio, and whether this needs to be addressed. It may be that finding ways to alleviate stress, perhaps through exercise and relaxation practices, can help you to cope with the demands of work. I also find that hypnotherapy (see page 206) helps a lot of women who get stressed very easily.

Men, too, often need to review their working patterns. Many men become defined by the work they do, and are ambitious to do it well, which is commendable but can sometimes be to the detriment of their lives. Often men feel that their role in conception is so minor, it doesn't matter if they continue to work as before. But 12-hour days, seven days a week, are incompatible with the demands of a young family, so it may be worth reviewing this now, too.

Many men feel very anxious about their role as breadwinner and provider, especially if there is the possibility of managing on only one salary for a while. This may make them feel that it is impossible to reduce their commitment to work, even if it is contributing to lack of success in getting pregnant in the first place.

Because of all of these demands, I spend a lot of time talking to couples about the issues arising from adjusting their work/life balance, and it is something I would suggest you take a long look at as part of your preparations to get pregnant.

Alcohol

Both men and women ask me all the time, 'How much should I drink?' Couples usually do not like to admit how much they really do drink. I generally advocate that a little of what you fancy does you good, but the research shows that in the four months leading up to conception, the chances of conceiving are far better if both partners avoid alcohol altogether. Studies have also shown that there is a definite link between miscarriage and alcohol consumption. For men, regular excessive drinking will affect sperm production. While the supposed 'safe' allowance is 14 units of alcohol a week for women, and 21 units for men, everyone is affected differently. Remember that a unit is the equivalent of one small glass of wine, a single measure of spirits, or half a pint of beer, lager or cider. It's not a huge amount, but even drinking this amount regularly will have an effect.

What concerns me are the high levels of drinking among professional couples, and particularly those high achievers who use alcohol to relax. I have one client who regularly drank 45 units or more a week, for example.

If someone is a regular drinker, cutting down or giving up can be quite difficult, especially for men, who often don't feel that it will significantly affect starting a family. Women, too, may be quite abstemious during their cycle, but the arrival of their period when they have been trying to conceive may make them hit the bottle in disappointment.

A couple of units a week really won't do any harm, but prior to any attempt to get pregnant I would advocate a week of complete abstinence for both partners (studies do show the effects leading up to ovulation – see page 167). Abstinence has the advantage of breaking the cycle of regular drinking, making it easier to cut down and to enjoy just the occasional glass of wine with a meal. When you don't drink you sleep better, eat better, and are generally more focused – all added advantages.

For many women who can't stop at a glass or two of wine, who tend to crave a drink at the end of the day and who drink every day, there is usually an underlying imbalance in their blood sugar. When there is fluctuating blood sugar – which can be exacerbated by drinking alcohol – it can result in a craving for alcohol, which provides a quick fix because of its sugar content. This can inadvertently fuel a cycle of binge drinking. Having a stable blood sugar level is so important for women, as explained in the Nutrition chapter, because of its effect on hormone production.

Answer these questions:

- Do you need something to get you going in the morning – tea, coffee or cigarettes?
- Do you have tea, coffee or cola at regular intervals during the day?
- Do you crave sweet foods?
- Do you have a high-carbohydrate, low-protein diet?
- Do you feel dizzy or irritable if you don't eat regularly?
- Do you often feel drowsy during the day?
- Are you unusually thirsty or hungry?
- Do you pass water frequently?

If you answer 'Yes' to most of these questions, it is a good indication that there is an imbalance in your blood sugar that needs to be addressed (see page 108). Women with low blood sugar tend to crave alcohol, and before you attempt to cut down or give up alcohol, it's important to correct the underlying blood sugar fluctuations, or hypo-glycaemia (low blood sugar). If you give up alcohol there is a tendency to have a huge craving for sweets, sugars and other simple carbohy-drates. This will tend to steer you back to alcohol.

The body's demand for sugar is partly fuelled by the brain's demand for serotonin, the feel-good hormone produced there. If your biochem-istry is naturally sugar-sensitive, you can easily get into the habit of drinking simply for the effect that the sugar/glucose has on your sero-tonin activity. Don't underestimate the power sugar has on the choices you make in your diet. If you are sugar-sensitive, sugar produces a similar euphoric high as opium or morphine. So you get a real rush, and the quest for that euphoric feeling will send you running out for a bar of chocolate, ice cream or an alcoholic drink – all of which are 'empty' calories with no nutrients of value, serving only to continue your blood sugar swings and their effect on your body and brain.

It's the destruction of the serotonin process that creates the intense cravings for sugar and alcohol. When you drink alcohol, your blood sugar spikes, and your body over-produces insulin to counteract the rise of blood sugar. But within 20 minutes or so, your blood sugar starts to plummet, and the serotonin effect starts to wear off. The brain has no reserves, and the demand creates the craving for the next drink and the next one.

When your blood sugar does drop, and isn't replaced, adrenaline is produced to counter the low glucose levels in the brain and body, which tricks the liver into releasing stored glycogen to prevent insulin shock. Insulin causes the cells in your body to absorb the glucose in your blood, which is why alcohol makes you feel so energetic – at least until the blood sugar drops again. But this blood sugar roller-coaster can only last as long as your adrenal glands are working, and not damaged.

Unsurprisingly, given the volatile nature of the body's biochemistry in reacting to and trying to accommodate all this, there is an impact on mood and feeling. Violent mood swings, explosive reactions, irritability and exhaustion are all features of unstable blood sugar levels.

The body produces, on average, an ounce of alcohol a day (equivalent to the amount in a glass and a half of wine or a pint of strong beer) from unused carbohydrates. A body that is constantly being fed excess amounts of sugar will produce even more. Alcohol produced in this way by the body, and alcohol that is drunk, are broken down by the body and converted to aceldehyde. Next it is converted to acetic acid (vinegar) and excreted from the body via the urine and the bile. If the liver can't keep up with the amount of aceldehyde produced, the aceldehyde is not effectively detoxed, and will find its way to the brain. It also means that the body remains in an acidic state, which is counter-productive to fertility (see page 113).

Problem drinkers tend to be very driven, high achievers, pleasure-seeking fun-lovers who actively seek out stimulating events. Not only that, but the sugar content of alcohol means that the bodies of regular drinkers get used to what is effectively a sugar rush for its energy. But high levels of simple carbohydrates don't provide the nutrients the body needs. While they provide an energy source of sorts, they don't provide it from a nutritional base. Simple carbohydrates are good for an emergency energy supply, and also stimulate the arousal, or 'fight or flight' response, which is exhausting both physically and mentally over the long term. As explained in the previous chapter, complex carbohydrates provide sustainable energy from a well-nourished body, keeping you calm and focused.

We also extract amino-acids from a balanced diet that includes protein, which produce the neurotransmitters necessary for proper brain activity. We need these neurotransmitters to regulate all our bodily functions, including our hormonal balance and control, so important for fertility. Drinking alcohol in excess can result in the sort of malnutrition that makes it impossible for the body to function properly in this way. A malnourished body finds it difficult to extract the nutrients you need, and equally finds it difficult to detox without the vitamins, minerals and amino acids it needs to do so.

Drinking too much alcohol also floods the body with free radicals. As explained on page 131, free radicals are very unstable and react quickly, trying to capture what they need to gain stability from other molecules. The 'attacked' molecule then loses its energy source, and becomes a free radical itself, beginning a chain reaction. Once the process is started, it can cascade, finally resulting in the disruption of living cells.

Alcohol is also well known for its disruption of the absorption and metabolism of B vitamins, so essential for fertility and hormonal balance. Without the B vitamins, which are water soluble and need to be accessed from the diet every day, other body functions are affected, including the synthesis of energy.

Alcohol disrupts the endocrine system, and is linked to hypothyroidism. It also destroys crucial enzymes in the body, which are essential for the digestion of proteins. Another problem with alcohol is that it makes the body excrete large amounts of zinc via the kidneys, which in turn disrupts the zinc/copper balance in the body.

Moderation is the key. Make sure you control what you drink and when, so that alcohol doesn't control you. Take a look at what triggers off a craving for a drink, and drink for pleasure, not for pain.

Smoking

There's no way round this one, really. If you want to get pregnant, you should stop smoking. Smoking reduces fertility in both women and men, and increases the length of time it takes to conceive. Women who smoke are twice as likely to be infertile as women who don't, and this is true for women attempting to get pregnant for the first time (primary infertility) and those who've already given birth before (secondary infertility). Research indicates that smoking may have an effect on the functioning of the Fallopian tubes.

Cigarette smoke contains nicotine, which is highly addictive, but that's not all. The US Government has approved 599 additives that are available to cigarette manufacturers, and cigarette smoke contains 4,000 different chemicals – many of which are highly toxic and cancer-causing. Among the many chemicals inhaled is carbon monoxide, and because this combines more readily than oxygen in the red blood cells, your body's oxygen intake is compromised. Oxidative stress, as it is called, is one of the major health hazards of smoking. Oxygen provides fuel to cell metabolism, so their function will be reduced without it – sperm production, for example, is affected by smoking. Men who smoke have a lower sperm count and a higher proportion of malformed sperm, while by-products of nicotine are found in the semen of smokers, which reduces the motility of sperm and affects their normal swimming patterns.

Smoking is an appetite suppressant, which means that the possibility of poor nutrition is increased. And as you know, good nutrition is vitally important to fertility. Smoking depletes your body of C and B vitamins, and allows for greater free radical damage. This explains why smokers age faster than non-smokers – and that's not just the visible signs of ageing, either. All cells, including the cell tissue of the ovaries and testes, will age more quickly than in non-smokers.

Evidence from numerous studies suggests that smoking affects the production of sex hormones in both men and women, and in women has been implicated with oestrogen deficiency and early menopause. Smokers are shown to have a reduced immune response, and smoking is also implicated in cervical cancer. Both nicotine and tobacco-specific carcinogens have been found in the cervical mucus of women who smoke.

Among couples undergoing IVF or other assisted conception methods, smokers are less likely to have a successful outcome. There seems to be some indication that the eggs of smokers are less likely to implant, and that smokers are more likely to suffer ectopic pregnancies and also to miscarry. Smoking affects the tiny hairs in the Fallopian tubes that waft the egg through the tube and towards the uterus.

Given the pervasive nature of the chemicals in cigarettes, and the effect of these on different body systems, it's hardly surprising that the toxicity has an effect on the reproductive cells of both men and women.

The very good news, however, is that giving up smoking can reverse its negative effects on fertility almost completely. Most studies show that women who were smokers but had stopped took no longer to conceive than women who had never smoked at all. With men, it takes up to three months for sperm quality and quantity to improve, but the degree of improvement can be significant.

There is no doubt that for a couple who smoke and are having difficulty conceiving, giving up is imperative. However, because of the highly addictive nature of nicotine, many find it very difficult although the desire to have a child and bring it up in a healthy environment, is quite a spur.

Techniques for giving up smoking

Avoid nicotine patches or chewing gum if you can, as keeping levels of nicotine in the body high is not good for fertility!

Start off by taking a quick look at what your 'triggers' are for cigarette smoking – for example:

- Do you smoke when talking on the telephone, when watching television or having a drink?
- Do you use cigarette smoking as a way of taking 'time out'?
- Do you smoke in the car?
- Do you smoke when under stress?
- Do you smoke before 10 a.m.?

Consider finding another activity to do at those times when you would automatically reach for a cigarette.

Many people find that cutting down before stopping helps to wean them off the addiction to nicotine. For example, never smoking before midday, then 6 p.m., or reducing their intake to a few a day. For others, going 'cold turkey' is the only way to break the pattern. Whatever you choose, you may find that your local health centre runs a Smoking Cessation clinic, which is worth checking out. Or contact Quitline, at www.quit.org.uk or on 0800 002200.

Hypnosis has proved invaluable to many people when giving up smoking. If you feel this might help, I would recommend it. Acupuncture, too, has helped many people. The biggest help, however, is actively wanting to stop. Ultimately, once your mind is convinced that you are no longer a smoker, the pull of the weed will lose its strength.

Drugs

Cannabis

I have seen numerous couples who smoke cannabis recreationally at weekends, and imagine that this occasional use will have no effect on their ability to conceive. Sadly, this is absolutely not the case. Research has shown that men in particular are adversely affected. While cannabis might be good for insomnia, glaucoma and multiple sclerosis, it isn't good for fertility. It contains around 400 active ingredients, of which perhaps the most potent is THC (tetrahydrocannabinol). While I have no opinion on whether or not cannabis should be legalized, I do know that adding to your toxic load is not conducive to fertility. Whether you smoke it, inhale it (through a bong) or eat it makes no difference. Cannabis is a powerful drug – like nicotine and alcohol – and ill advised if you and your partner are trying to conceive.

Cocaine

Again, I see couples who use cocaine recreationally and feel that doing so at weekends is fine. Cocaine is an extremely powerful stimulant that raises the heart rate and body temperature, and suppresses the appetite. It is highly addictive, the 'hit' only lasts for 20-30 minutes, and coming down can increase feelings of depression, so the temptation to take more tends to increase. Frequent use tends to repress sexual desire and after a heavy bout can leave you feeling as if you've got a dose of flu. None of which is great if you are trying to have a baby.

Medications that affect fertility

It's also worth considering those medicines – prescription and non-prescription – that may be inadvisable while trying to get pregnant. For example, some painkillers are anti-spasmodics, which may actually prevent ovulation. Other drugs may not have such a dire effect, but may dry up mucus secretions (as is the case with anti-histamines), and this will reduce the amount of cervical secretions produced.

While trying to get pregnant, it's probably as well to avoid the following, which can have an effect on cervical mucus, ovulation or sperm count:

- Acne treatments – The prescription drug Accutane shouldn't be taken, as it has been linked to foetal abnormalities.
- NSAIDs (non-steroidal anti-inflammatory) painkillers, such as ibuprofen – These should be used infrequently. Heavy use can interfere with ovulation. Use paracetamol instead.
- Anti-depressants – Drugs such as serotonin re-uptake inhibitors have an effect on brain chemistry, which may also affect hormone balance.
- Anti-malarial pills – These have been linked to foetal abnormalities and should be out of your system for at least three months before you conceive. Some schools of thought recommend even longer than this. So keep this in mind if you are travelling anywhere that requires you to take anti-malaria pills. Some research has been done on the herbal treatment Artemisia as an anti-malarial, but there is no guarantee that this is a truly effective alternative.
- Anti-histamines – Cough medicines are designed to dry up mucus secretions, and should be avoided. Remember that vitamin C is also an anti-histamine and shouldn't be taken in doses larger than 1,000 mg while trying to conceive.
- Steroids – Cortisone and prednisolone are the most common, and

can be found in inhalers, too. In high enough doses they will affect the pituitary gland, possibly inhibiting the hormone secretion necessary for ovulation.

- Antibiotics – If you are prescribed these, mention to your doctor that you are trying for a baby, as some varieties can affect sperm production.
- Diuretics – These can have an effect on cervical mucus secretion.

A Quick Checklist of Medicines to Avoid If You Are Trying to Conceive

- antibiotics
- anti-depressants
- anti-histamines
- anti-hypertensives
- anti-malarial pills
- antiviral drugs
- decongestants
- inhalers
- NSAID painkillers
- sleeping pills
- steroids

Environmental Impact on Fertility

The environment in which you work can play a part in your fertility, too. Environmental factors are being blamed for the reduction of the male sperm count, which has fallen considerably over the last 20 years. Chemicals, plastics, exhaust fumes, pesticides – our day-to-day environment is filled with substances that can harm us, including our fertility.

Chemicals at home and in the workplace

Working with chemicals, for example in printing or hairdressing, may be a contributory factor. Just be aware if you are using any chemicals in your profession (or in any hobbies you pursue) such as solvents, dyes, etc., and take measures to reduce the risks by using the proper protective equipment – masks, gloves, etc. – regularly.

Be aware, too, that just because a chemical occurs naturally in the environment doesn't mean it is safe. One example of this is isoflavones found in foods such as soybeans, which have an oestrogen-like effect and should not be consumed in large amounts.

In the home, choose carefully when shopping for air-fresheners, oven-cleaners and the like.

Cosmetics and toiletries

Attention is also being turned to those chemicals that are routinely used in toiletries, personal hygiene and beauty care products, from preservatives in moisturizers to formaldehyde in nail polish hardeners, because of their possible toxicity. For example, wearing nail polish regularly leads to the absorption of a certain amount of formaldehyde, because our nails are porous. This may not cause a reaction, but formaldehyde is highly toxic, a carcinogen, neurotoxic and genotoxic (can affect genetic material) and over time may place an additional demand on the liver, the body's organ of detoxification, depleting your natural resources and ability to keep the body clear of toxins.

Although most chemicals in regular use do not pose a big threat, the incessant exposure to one or more products over long periods of time can create problems.

In the same way that we became more conscious of chemical additives and preservatives finding their way into our foods, many people are taking to checking the labels on their personal hygiene and beauty products, from moisturizers, shaving creams, sun-protection, deodorants, toothpaste, panty liners, nail polish removers and talcum powder to tampons, retinol creams and hair dyes. As a rule of thumb, the more chemical ingredients listed on the product's contents, the better it is to avoid it. For a checklist of products that could do harm, and alter-natives, please visit the Women's Environmental Network site (www.wen.org.uk).

Happily, as more and more consumers are becoming aware of the dangers and demanding alternatives, the range of safe and organic products is increasing all the time.

Remember, though, that it's important to be aware that even herbal remedies and other 'natural' products can affect fertility. St John's Wort, for example, inhibits sperm motility, while echinacea interferes with sperm enzymes.

Electromagnetic fields

I am often asked about whether or not mobile phones are dangerous, and whether or not they should be avoided. As most of us now own a mobile phone and use it regularly, it's not surprising that the question gets raised. The official line is that mobile phone technology isn't new, and has been studied for the last 60 years, and shows no sign of causing damage. The alternative view is that we are increasingly exposed to levels of electromagnetic radiation, from phones and other sources, and that the pulsed microwaves from mobile phones constitute an electromagnetic hazard that has been linked to a range of illnesses, from headaches to memory loss.

There is research to show that mobile phones affect fertility. Be careful about carrying a phone in your pocket.

My view is to err on the side of caution. Using a mobile phone endlessly, day in and day out, is probably best avoided. I have come across no hard evidence to suggest that mobile phones are detrimental to fertility, but it may be that the research has not yet been done. In the meantime, use only when necessary, and don't carry it on your person.

A word, here, too, about laptops. These also emit electromagnetic waves, and you should avoid actually sitting it on your lap as you go about your work.

Stress

I see countless women worrying that they are too stressed to conceive. People use the word 'stress' very easily. I feel that if you get the control back in your life, the stress will sort itself out.

It is all very well being told to 'chill' and conception will happen. When it doesn't, you get stressed, your thoughts and conversations are about babies and everyone around you seems to be pregnant. I know that you want to feel you are being pro-active, but you need to deal with your 'internal' environment. The mind/body connection is so important. Taking into account the mental well-being of couples suffering from fertility problems is so vital in the work that I do. Most women have lost faith in their bodies to do the right thing. The body is always trying to do the right thing, it is always trying to achieve homeostasis (the body's natural balance).

Case History: Ruth

Ruth was 36 and had been trying for a baby for three years. A busy university lecturer, teaching PhD students all day, she spent time not only helping them with their studies but sorting out their personal lives and being like a mother to them. This was eating into her home time. Also she had an elderly mother who was in

---

poor health. Most evenings were spent marking, lecture-planning and answering her emails. Ruth was completely in her head, thinking all of the time, giving out emotionally to everyone else but leaving nothing for herself. When eventually she did go to bed, she read books, crime and murder novels, so her head was full of yet more thoughts. She felt duty-bound by everything and could not say no.

The priority for Ruth was to build up her reserves, rest more and get the information overload out of her head. We organized sessions of meditation and deep breathing. No more reading crime novels late at night before sleep. I also helped her to plan how to reduce the hours she spent marking papers and spend more time together with her partner. She had to train herself to be supportive of her students but not immersed in their problems. I also advised her to aim to get to bed by 10.30 p.m. and to have a massage once every two weeks. She also needed to learn to make more time for herself rather than other people.

The Brain and Stress

Consider what your brain has to do every day, masterminding every move, decision, emotion or action you take. It often runs on empty because you've got up late and have had no time for a nutritious breakfast. It is often fuelled by caffeine and nicotine, and bombarded by stimuli like noise and air pollution, lights that are too bright, fluctuating stress hormones and more. It works for extended hours without adequate rest, and is bathed in stress hormones that are, in themselves, neurotoxins. And in our 24-hour society, the brain seldom gets any time off to recharge properly. Faced with this sort of biochemical challenge, is it any wonder that the pituitary gland, situated deep in the brain, is negatively affected?

One of the key messages I want to emphasize is that learning to manage stress is crucial if you want to maximize your chances of conceiving successfully. Your brain has to process and adjust to stimuli – visual, auditory, chemical – constantly, and if you don't allow time for it to download and recharge, it will suffer. Learning how to discharge emotions, relax, meditate, sleep soundly, breathe properly – all of this helps the brain to restore itself and function properly – and this includes balancing its hormonal output.

Case History: Hannah

Hannah was in her early 30s, a high achiever. She worked long hours as a trader – getting up at 5.30 and working through to 9 at night. She started the day on no breakfast – an adrenaline junkie – instead using sugar, alcohol and caffeine to keep her going. She was also obsessed with her weight.

Hannah was earning a fortune in bonuses and had control over most areas of her life; pregnancy was the only thing that was eluding her. She would come into the office on her mobile and manage to be rude to reception staff, upsetting everything in her wake.

Hannah was keen to undertake my whole programme of acupuncture, nutrition – the works. She wanted the solutions and was convinced, if she threw enough money at it, the problem would go away. What she was not willing to do, however, was change. She wanted a nutritional consultation, but she was not going to eat breakfast or give up coffee. In Chinese Medicine terms, the way I work, she was a Wood type person: very angry, aggressive and completely out of control (see page 226 for more about different 'types' in Traditional Chinese Medicine).

To her horror, I would not let Hannah do any of the pro-grammes – she thought if she was paying, she could choose to do whatever she wanted. Eventually she did come back – she started to eat breakfast and, over a four-week period – we cut out sugar and alcohol, and got Hannah to take a walk in the fresh air three days a week. We never quite got round to reducing her hours, but got her to have sex more frequently and she did conceive.

Many of my clients are driven by high expectations of results and rewards, which they achieve by, often, quite fanatical levels of control and commitment. They expect it in others as well as themselves, and almost need to be 'given permission' to slow down. Allowing them to give this permission to themselves is one of the crucial objectives of my clinic's programme. So many women feel unfulfilled and not proactive in their pursuit of getting pregnant unless they are having endless treatments and appointments. For some couples who come to the clinic wanting to do the whole programme, it comes as a shock when I say no, we are doing nothing. I do not want you to have more appointments – I want you to have a break. I often encourage them to go and learn to meditate, come off the Internet, have a massage regularly, drink a glass of wine, watch TV in the morning, eat an ice cream, stay in bed until 11 on a Sunday reading the papers.

Case History: Tamara

Tamara was a busy PR consultant who came along to the clinic after having tried unsuccessfully for two years to get pregnant. We organized one fertility awareness session for her plus one nutrition session and a course of four sessions of acupuncture to regulate her menstrual cycle. She came into the clinic one day very stressed, as she felt she was doing too much. I sat down with her and went through the treatments she was having. What I hadn't realized was that, on top of what she was doing at my clinic, on a weekly basis she was also going elsewhere and having reflexology, osteopathy, taking Chinese herbs and having counselling – no wonder she was stressed! I talked with her about which of the treatments she was having made her feel the most relaxed. It turned out it was the reflexology. So I tried to encourage her to stick with this. She had not liked the acupuncture as she hated needles, but thought if it hurt it was doing her good. The Chinese herbs she was taking were not only making her gag, they were costing her a lot of money. I told her to stop taking them. It is so hard to persuade, especially women, that they are doing too much and just need to keep it simple and focused. Many feel that doing something, anything, is better than doing nothing.

Balancing stress and your internal environment

Mind over body – we all quote this, but do we ever really consider our internal environment and the effect of stress on our everyday lives? It wreaks havoc on our hormones and our immune systems, all the body systems are working flat out trying to achieve balance. There is enough evidence to show the effect of our emotions on reproduction. Very often couples are predominant in one emotion: worry, fear, anger, grief. This can affect the body's inner networks. Acupuncture can rebalance this.

Stress happens every day in our lives. If you are trying to conceive, these stresses can include 'Will the test be positive?' 'Will I have another miscarriage?' 'How will I cope if the IVF is not successful this time?' 'What if I never get pregnant?' This kind of continual worry, fear, anger and grief affect the hormones and weaken the system.

It is not acute stress that affects us most, but the chronic kind.

'How do I know if I am stressed or out of balance?' – some of you will be reading this in a panic. You need to look at your lifestyle and try and work out ways of getting the balance back. If you are working long hours but enjoy your job, this is positive, but what goes with long hours tends to be a poor diet and poor eating habits, lack of sleep and no sex, usually. So look at cutting down. If you do not like your job, think about changing it. Other stress factors can be financial worries, the death of a relative, your relationship with your parents, stepchildren, ex-husband or ex-wife. All of these carry emotions, often very negative ones. But the positive thing is, the body has an amazing ability to counter the effects of stress. This is simply called relaxation: deep breathing, meditation, sleep. These things help you to turn off all of the warning bells and reduce stress and tension.

Everyone feels stressed at one time or another. A degree of stress is an inevitable part of life, but it's when it becomes a constant feature of daily life that problems arise. Stress is a particularly insidious state; it creeps up on you until you don't realize that your muscles are permanently tense, your heart rate is constantly raised and your breathing is shallow. All are typical physical symptoms of the stress response, when the sympathetic nervous systems secretes the hormones adrenaline and cortical to rev us up for a potential 'fight or flight'.

Where fight or flight is needed, this response is perfect. However, when this becomes a constant, learned response to life, these raised hormone levels begin to feel 'normal' – taking a toll on our physical health and putting other body systems out of balance.

Long-term low levels of stress are exhausting. This state of permanent arousal automatically makes us feel anxious rather than energized, and that can lead to depression. Stress-induced anxiety can also make us prone to panic attacks – where the symptoms can actually be quite scary. A pounding heart, pain in the chest, difficulty breathing, tingling sensations in the limbs – symptoms such as these can lead people to believe they are having a heart attack.

The hormones secreted to sustain this state were never intended to be constantly circulating in the body, and when they do they are really quite toxic to various body systems – the brain, the endocrine system and the immune system. This constant heightened state also makes it difficult to relax, and to sleep. This in turn increases the stress under which the body is placed. It's another vicious circle.

The additional toxic load that stress places on the body also needs detoxifying. The constant production and detoxifying of these hormones places demands on the body that need to be met nutritionally, and this in turn diverts nutritional resources away from other body systems, like the reproductive system.

If you answer yes to any of the questions below, there's a sustained level of chronic stress in your life that needs to be addressed:

- Do you find it difficult to get off to sleep?
- Do you wake during the night?
- Do you wake during the early hours of the morning, and can't get back to sleep again?
- Do you find it difficult to relax when you have time off?
- Do you find yourself fidgety and restless when you do have time off?
- Do you suffer indigestion?
- Do you have a permanent sensation of mild nausea?
- Do you crave coffee and other stimulants?
- Do you find yourself forgetting things you've just gone to get?
- Do you find yourself snappy and irritable?
- Are you prone to tearfulness?

For more about stress and its effect on your brain, see the Nutrition chapter.

Building Up Your Reserves

Exercise

In Chinese Medicine you build up your reserves of energy with sleep, meditation and t'ai chi or qi gong exercise. The Chinese use qi gong and t'ai chi to strengthen the system and focus the breath, meditation to discharge, renew and relax the brain, and sleep to renew and recharge your batteries.

I am often asked 'How much exercise should I take?' 'When in my cycle should I exercise?' 'Should I stop exercising after ovulation?' I think very often the answer to these questions depends on the type of exercise you are doing, plus your body weight.

Exercise can help with problems such as PCOS, where it can be a fun and enjoyable way to maintain a healthy weight and control insulin levels. And enjoying the exercise you do is important. It is no good forcing yourself to go to the gym if you hate it. Doing exercise you enjoy – dancing, walking, swimming – is far more beneficial. I feel that many of the women I see are exercising far too much (exercising for more than 15 hours a week may affect and inhibit ovulation), and I encourage them to cut down. Exercise in moderation – no more than three aerobic sessions a week – is good for endorphin-release and can prevent depression.

Our bodies are built for movement. The musculo-skeletal system remains strong, and supports the other body systems. Without strong muscles, other organs suffer.

Most of us lead very sedentary lives, without enough regular exercise, and everything from our breathing (and oxygen levels) to our lymphatic circulation (and detoxification) is negatively affected by the lack of activity in our lives.

Fortunately, this can be rectified quite simply. If you take a 20-minute walk three times a week, you will notice an improvement in your muscle tone and mood after only a month. This may not be enough, but it's a good start! Try to choose something that you enjoy, either alone or with friends, so you will do it regularly, whether it's playing badminton or joining a yoga class.

A word here about swimming. A lot of my clients ask me about the benefits of swimming, and in all honesty I tell them that, while it is a great form of exercise, the chlorine in pools can have a negative effect on fertility. But so long as you try not to ingest a lot of chlorine while you swim (try keeping your head out of the water as much as you can), if you enjoy swimming then you should do it.

Whatever you choose, do remember not to overdo it. I sometimes see couples who have become fanatical about exercise, to the point where they are rigorously exercising every day. While they may be achieving levels of undreamed-of fitness, there is evidence to show that excessive exercise has an impact on fertility hormone levels. Sperm production can decrease, and in some women the fertility hormones are suppressed to the point where ovulation ceases. As with all things, balance is key.

Relaxation

Ask many people how they relax, and they will look blankly at you! It can be hard for some people really to relax, but simple things – a walk, watching a film, reading – can all help. Many of us have come to feel there's no time in a busy schedule for relaxation, and the process of driving relentlessly on has become habitual. It actually becomes such a way of life that it becomes familiar, even comfortable. Then, when the pressure is off, we actually feel uncomfortable – so we consciously choose to return to it. Lack of relaxation is a common 21st-century problem which demands resistance for the sake of our health. Constant tension causes physical problems, from raised blood pressure to irritable bowel syndrome. Our bodies feel the stress of the tension in our muscles, and this serves to make us feel emotionally stressed, too. It's a vicious circle and it's insidious: it creeps up on you until you are living in such a state of tension it begins to feel normal.

Muscular tension, which occurs automatically when we live in constant stress because of the production of hormones like adrenaline and corticosteroids, has an inhibiting effect on relaxation. Sometimes it gets to the point when the muscular tension is so locked in it becomes impossible to shift without external help, like a massage. Bear this in mind and try to avoid it happening by incorporating some regular exercise into your daily life to loosen up your muscles.

You can include relaxation techniques in your breathing exercises (see page 186). These help you differentiate between tense and relaxed muscles, which will help your muscles 'relearn' the relaxed state. Tense muscles do not get enough blood flow or oxygen, making them susceptible to damage – and damage to the structures they are supposed to support, like the neck, shoulders and spine. Lack of adequate oxygen also makes muscles produce lots of lactic acid. An acidic state within the body isn't healthy. High levels of lactic acid places additional strain on the liver, too. The liver converts lactic acid, or lactate, to glucose for energy – which contributes to the body's sense that it should be doing some physical exercise! Persistently high levels of lactic acid can also contribute to chronic fatigue syndrome.

For many who have functioned with high levels of stress for a while, learning to relax takes time, and may even involve some sort of physical activity beforehand to free up tense muscles. For others it means taking a long hot bath by candlelight, listening to music, immersing themselves in a good book or taking a solitary walk. What is important is to find something that works for you, and integrate it into your daily life.

Where stress has become so problematic some help is needed. Hypnotherapy can be of great value (see page 206). Many couples having problems getting pregnant are easily recognizable as high-achieving and stressed-out, and they benefit from some guided thera-py to help them relearn patterns of relaxation. Set yourself a goal of 20 minutes a day.

Breathing

We all do it automatically, from the moment of birth until we die. But breathing is both automatic and something we can influence at will, and because of the mind/body link we have a powerful tool at our fin-gertips. We can learn to breathe in a way that influences our physical, psychological and spiritual well-being. Just by breathing in a mindful, focused way clears the head of other thoughts.

Most of us breathe very shallowly, using the top part of the chest. This creates tension that radiates up into our shoulders, neck muscles, fore-head and face, and also restricts the internal organs of the abdomen.

The good news is that we can learn to breathe in a way that relieves tension and stress, raises internal oxygen levels and creates a relaxed state. Breathing diaphragmatically, as we were designed to do, also means that the diaphragm stops being a tight ring around the aorta, so should reduce blood pressure, and also allows the large colon under-neath the diaphragm to be gently massaged rather than constricted, which helps to reduce tension in the gut. According to many experts, learning to breathe properly is the most important tool available for stress-management.

Breathing Exercise

1. Lie on your back with your knees bent so your back is comfortably flat on the floor without strain.
2. Consciously relax your shoulders and tuck your chin in so your neck is lengthened. A small cushion under your head is fine.
3. Gently rest one hand on your upper chest and one on your abdomen.
4. Close your eyes and breathe gently and regularly in through your nose and out through your mouth.
5. Notice your chest rising and, on each breath, take it a little deeper into your abdomen so you can feel your ribs expand slightly and your abdomen extend.
6. Place your hands by your sides and continue breathing in this way.
7. As your breathing becomes calmer and more efficient, you should find that you are breathing in and out, naturally, between 12 and 16 times a minute, less as you really relax.

Practise this for 10 minutes two or three times a day, until this new way of breathing becomes automatic whether you are lying down, sitting or standing.

Sometimes it's helpful to silently intone the word 'in' on the in-breath, and 'out' on the out-breath. It sounds obvious, but is actually quite helpful in keeping your mind focused on your breathing.

If a breathing exercise isn't enough to stop your thoughts crowding in, try imagining yourself as a pebble, dropping into a pool of water, dropping down and down through the still, cool depths. Using visualization such as this helps many people learn how to relax.

Visualization

Visualization means imagining yourself somewhere where you feel safe, secure and peaceful. This takes practice; many people find it difficult at first, but it becomes easier over time.

Imagine somewhere – maybe a lovely, warm sandy beach where all you can hear is the gentle lapping of the waves, or a beautiful woodland walk where dappled sunlight falls through the leaves, the air is soft and the only sound is occasional bird song – choose whatever works for you.

After taking your breathing to a gentle level, as described above, take yourself to this place in your imagination. Experience it, in your imagination, through your senses. Do you feel warm? Imagine the sun's rays gently penetrating your clothes, warming your skin. What sounds can you hear? What can you see in your mind's eye? By concentrating on your physical sensations as you take yourself through this visualized space, you free your conscious mind from the bombardment of other stimuli.

Not only is visualization relaxing, it can help tremendously if you use it to envisage the future and outcomes you want. Our minds are very receptive to this kind of positive thinking. I sometimes encourage couples to use visualization to 'see' the fertilized embryo travelling down to the uterus and safely implanting there, for example.

(For more about visualization, see page 209 in the next chapter.)

Meditation

I made it my goal this year to learn to meditate. I never thought I would be able to achieve this, as I have never been able to clear all the thoughts from my head. The beauty of the meditation I was taught was that you do not have to. No matter what thoughts come into your head, you accept them and do not try to avoid them, but just keep repeating a sound that you are given. By repeating the sound, tension is released. This is also a great way to discharge the negative emotions of the day. I learned with a group called ACEM and the training does not cost a fortune, around £80–£100.

Meditation used to be thought of as the 'flaky' side of Eastern mysticism, and a lot of people were deeply sceptical about it. What we now know is that those who learn to meditate are really on to something – not least allowing the emergence of alpha brain waves to help them utilize their brain's power more adequately, while also reducing the inhibiting effects of stress on both the mind and body.

Meditation is a learned skill for most of us. It takes an initial practice of around 10 to 15 minutes a day and, like a lot of skills, some people find it easier to master than others. For many, finding a weekend course of instruction, or a retreat, can often be a good start, but it's not essential. You can learn to meditate alone, in your own home.

Preparing for meditation includes getting comfortable and utilizing a calming pattern of breathing (see page 186). The idea is to reduce your brain's activity consciously – allowing alpha waves to predominate. You do this by allowing any thought processes to simply come and go without examination.

Few people find this easy! We are so geared up to thinking about the next thing we have to do, even while doing something else, that our brains are constantly in a state of anticipation. This comes to feel normal. Many people find that focusing on an object, like a candle flame, working our way through the breathing and relaxation exercises in preparation, or constantly repeating a phrase or word, a mantra, helps. Finally, these unwelcome intrusions on our thoughts just fail to register, and we are meditating!

Sleep

I am always going on about the importance of sleep to my clients. So many of them wake in the early hours of the morning worrying about whether they are going to have a baby or not. This is always the worst time of day.

We don't just fall asleep and stay solidly asleep for six, seven or eight hours. We sleep in cycles of changing brain activity, and while our bodies can just about manage physically with little or no sleep over a period of time, our brains can't. Switching off conscious brain activity, through sleep, is essential for brain health and proper functioning.

We all have an internal 'body clock' that functions roughly on a 24-hour cycle. This cycle is also referred to as the circadian rhythm, and it governs the cycle of bodily functions: at what times you feel sleepy or wakeful, energized or tired, when you want to eat, and fluctuations in body temperature and hormone secretion.

In fact our natural circadian rhythm is closer to 25 hours than 24, but we maintain the 24-hour cycle through a process of constant readjustment. Knowing when the fluctuations of our daily cycle occur means we can work with them rather than against them. For example, there is a natural energy surge in the morning, which peaks at around 11 a.m. It then dips at around 3 p.m., roughly eight hours after waking and approximately halfway through a day's activity. For many, this is the optimum time for a nap, to recharge for the remainder of the day and to guard *against* extreme exhaustion before bedtime. Going to bed *before* you are completely exhausted actually helps you sleep better: it allows time to relax, switch off and achieve better sleep!

These rhythms are partly learned, which is why we can change them or adjust to different time zones. But we are diurnal creatures, as opposed to nocturnal, meaning that we are geared to function during daylight hours and sleeping when it is dark. This process is influenced most by the hormone melatonin, secreted by the pineal gland. It is the secretion of melatonin, which is a derivative of serotonin, a hormone responsible for influencing mood, that maintains our day and night pattern. The secretion of melatonin increases in response to the reduced light at night, helping us to sleep, and it can be taken in pill form to help induce sleep in people who suffer from insomnia. We know, for example, that secretion of this hormone decreases as we age – one reason that elderly people often find it difficult to sleep well, or soundly, at night.

Hormone secretions also control temperature fluctuation. For example, your temperature begins to drop towards its daily minimum as you fall asleep at the end of the day, and begins to peak again as you wake. Levels of corticosteroids diminish towards the end of the day, and build to a high level just before you wake. This explains why you feel the cold more when you are very tired and how, through inadequate amounts of sleep, you can over-produce 'awake' hormones to compensate. In order to maintain well-functioning circadian rhythms, what our bodies really like is regularity.

Tips to help you sleep

- Have a consistent bed time.
- Get up at the same time every day.
- Try going to bed 15 minutes earlier each night and see how you feel the next day.
- Keep your bedroom dark and quiet.
- Don't watch television in the bedroom.
- If you cannot fall asleep within 30 minutes, get up for a bit.
- Avoid caffeine and alcohol at night.

thoughts and emotions

One of the questions I ask all of my clients is, 'Is there anything happening psychologically or emotionally for you that could actually be stopping you from getting pregnant?' You shouldn't have to dig too deep to come up with an answer, nor have anybody put suggestions to you. Most women will know if there is something lurking in the background.

It's obvious to me that enabling my clients to deal with their emotions helps them to get through the process. Most Western medicine is (quite rightly) concerned with sorting out issues on a physical level, but I like to take a look at the whole picture: the grief, the anger, the frustration, the guilt and the laughter are all part of what I share every day. Using treatments to help women sort their emotions as important as the physical investigations.

Our thoughts and the way we think determine our emotional and physical state. I feel that negativity and negative thoughts can, at some level, act as a block when trying for a baby. Now, I don't want anyone reading this to panic suddenly and think, 'Oh my God, I am so negative I am never going to conceive!' This chapter is able to help you let go and understand how you can change from being negative to positive and how to deal with some of the emotions you may be feeling.

I have found hypnotherapy to be a really useful tool to help clients restructure negative thought patterns and emotions, and will refer to this specifically.

In Chinese medicine thoughts are energy, waiting to be used skilfully through our emotions. To the Chinese, different emotions affect different organs and can weaken and block the energy flow around the body. While it is appropriate to feel anger, frustration, grief, etc., it is being able to manage these emotions and understand and let go of them that is important for health. Many women are unaware of the potential they have within to change things, instead looking constantly outside themselves for answers.

First of all, you need to acknowledge these thoughts:

• Try to identify the cause of your negative thinking and how long these kinds of thoughts have been with you.
• Try and think back to where you first heard them: mother, family member, teacher, etc.
• Do these thoughts cause you stress?
• Try to look at people around you, how they react to you.
• Try and look at outcomes: if the situation were to change from a negative to a positive, how would you really feel?

Whenever you work towards supporting yourself physically – through improved diet, gentle exercise, better relaxation, and improved sleep – how you feel emotionally will also improve.

There's no question about it: Your emotional health may on some level affect your ability to conceive. While it is perfectly normal to experience anger, fear, worry and grief, when these emotions take over everything else, blocking you, problems can arise.

Trying for a baby is inevitably a very emotional time for couples and stressful to your relationship. There is no doubt that, whether or not there are problems conceiving, pregnancy, birth and early parenthood challenge even the most secure of relationships. Not only that, but when you try to become a parent, and succeed, there are consequences for all your relationships. In most cases these are positive, but they can be complex and occasionally negative.

It's easy, when focusing on the physical, to underestimate the impact on your emotional life. If you are someone who has always been very fit and healthy, you may feel perplexed and angry if you fail to get pregnant. If you are someone who is used to getting what you want, whether by dint of hard work or luck, and what you want isn't happening, it's easy to get upset and disillusioned. And, being only human, these uncomfortable and distressing feelings have an impact on the people closest to us.

Although with fertility the emphasis is often on the woman, it is also difficult, emotionally, for men. A man may feel powerless in the face of his partner's desire to get pregnant, willing to help but not sure how. He may also feel that the focus of the relationship has changed from the close intimacy of being a couple, where his needs were considered important, to being relegated to mere stud value. The desire for a baby can become dominant in a relationship, and sometimes this obscures what the primary motive for starting a family was all about.

I try to help the couples I see get the balance back in the relationship, helping them to feel positive about one another, positive about the decisions they have made, positive about moving on and feeling secure about where they are going. Men do find it very hard to express their emotions. When you ask a woman how she feels, she will talk endlessly. When you ask a man, the response is usually one word: 'Fine.' Many men can be very defensive, resenting the endless therapies their partners are going through in pursuit of a baby. A woman, on the other hand, may complain, 'I've given up everything; he's not trying hard enough.' My response is always the same: Be kind to one another; remember what you had before all this started.

Trying to start a family often raises long-buried issues for couples – issues that may be linked to past family experiences, traumatic or otherwise – and expectations and anxieties about what sort of parents you'll be, balancing family and work or the pressures of being the main breadwinner. These can resonate at a deep level and may not surface until a couple are facing problems with conception. Being aware of where some of your emotions are rooted can help in understanding why you feel as you do, and lessening the impact. A lot of couples do feel close when they are trying for a baby or going through IVF, but will inevitably reach a crisis point, and one that may be different for each of you.

One factor that has an influence on a couple's thinking and approach to conception is age, particularly the age of the woman, and this can bring its own anxiety. Women tend to get into panic mode. The reasons for failing to conceive straight away are covered elsewhere in this book; what I'm concerned about here are the emotions that go along with it.

What we know is that there are some fairly standard emotional reactions to failing to conceive straight away. These emotions are commonly expressed by both women and men who come to see me, and include:

- guilt
- grief – 'I may never achieve the one thing in life I've always wanted.'
- isolation – 'All my friends have children and I don't fit in any more.'
- fear – 'What if I *never* get pregnant?'
- frustration – 'Why am I having problems when everyone else seems to manage to get pregnant?'
- anger – 'It's not fair.'
- shock – 'I never expected this to happen to me.'
- apprehension – 'What happens next?' 'Will I be able to cope?'
- anxiety – 'If I need fertility treatment, how can we afford it?'
- denial – 'This can't be happening to me.'
- responsibility – 'I feel I've let my partner and family down.'
- failure – 'There's something wrong with me.'

- envy – 'I feel jealous and don't want to spend time with friends with babies.'
- regret – 'Perhaps I've left it too late.'
- depression.

For some people, expressing their feelings comes easily. For others, repressing them actually feels easier, but this is unhelpful. It's important to talk through with your partner, without recrimination, how you feel. It's also important to explain to your wider family – especially if they are constantly asking 'So when are you going to make me a grandmother, then?' – what the situation is. Keep it simple.

Friends, too, will probably be more supportive than you think. It can also be very helpful to see a trained counsellor. I recommend this to many couples who have got stuck in their different emotional states and are finding communicating with each other difficult. This helps weed out the emotions from the facts, and helps identify what is causing the most distress, and alleviating it.

Guilt

Guilt covers a wide range of emotions. The most common problem is around past terminations, where women feel very guilty about a decision they made years ago. They may be harbouring a feeling that God is now punishing them, that the previous pregnancy was their only chance and they blew it. There may, as another example, be guilt around a previous affair by either partner. Many have told their partners all about it and are working through it all, but are still left with the feeling that they don't 'deserve' to have a baby because of what they have done. Very often the relief when a woman sits and tells me is huge, as they have been carrying this burden around for months.

Carrie, 35, was not getting pregnant and her relationship was starting to deteriorate. She found herself becoming attracted to someone single and younger at work. Flirting with this man made her feel attractive again, which she hadn't done for months. Then, remorse hit her.

Hypnosis helped Carrie explore the situation and off-load the guilt without endangering her stable relationship.

At our clinic we try to help women come to terms with all kinds of past decisions, to recognize and deal with guilt constructively, forgive themselves and begin to generate a positive expectation of becoming a parent. In the case of a woman who has had a termination in the past, for example, we try to help them to see, that the positive side of this past decision is that it proves they can get pregnant. This is the foundation that we build from.

Other issues are the impact on some men if their current partner, or even a previous partner, has had a termination with them in the past. They are unable to have sex because on a deep level they remain frightened of getting them pregnant.

Very often women don't tell their partner if they have had a termination in the past and are terrified of their partner finding out. I always encourage them to be open and honest, as I believe that a lack of this kind of communication causes emotional blocks.

Performance Anxiety

Performance anxiety is very common. It can become a major stumbling block on the road to conception. There is almost a Catch-22 scenario where the male partner needs to 'perform' to impregnate his partner, but the pressure of 'on-the-spot sex' at specific times of the month can make a man's libido and basic equipment unresponsive. This situation can add further pressure on an already fraught situation if the woman believes that her partner is somehow not as committed as she is to conception. Blame can set in and relationships can be stretched to breaking point. Remember, it's nobody's fault that it hasn't happened yet. Don't get into recriminations like 'I know you don't want a baby as much as me.'

Second-time relationships

There are undoubtedly all kinds of stresses and emotional baggage around second-time relationships. Having to look after other people's children, step-children visiting at weekends, no time for intimacy, vengeful ex-partners, resentment about alimony, acrimonious divorces – they all take their toll emotionally. How you deal with this can make a huge difference to how you feel. You have to let go of the anger, grief, frustration and resentment or it will eat away at you and your relationship.

These situations are becoming more common. A woman whose partner has children from a previous relationship can sometimes feel that her man is not as committed as she is, because this will, for him, be just another child. There are very often additional stress factors such as finance, a partner's ex-wife or ex-husband, etc. Many women blame their difficulties being able to conceive on the stress all these factors bring.

Miriam, 37, resented the fact that her husband's 4-year-old child lived with them for half of the week. She felt that this child was undisciplined and spoilt; she felt jealous of the time her partner spent with him, and resented looking after him when her partner was not home. It's hard to feel good about these kinds of feelings: Miriam knew she shouldn't feel this way. At the same time, she felt that since her husband had a child already he wasn't as bothered about having another. The relationship really started to suffer, as Miriam felt herself becoming more and more negative.

First off, Miriam had to acknowledge that, yes, she was in fact jealous of this child. And we reassured her that it is very difficult looking after somebody else's child. She had chosen this relationship and had fully committed that she would accept the child. She had been idealistic about what having a child age 4 would be like. We helped her, through hypnosis, to understand how her partner was feeling, and how hard it must be for him trying to please everyone.

Once she was able to accept her feelings, she was free to work on ways of improving the situation. This meant getting a better relationship with the child and learning more about how her behaviour was probably affecting the way the child behaved. She also started to explore ways she could discuss the situation and her feelings with her partner in a way that wouldn't be confrontational or lead to rows, but would be productive for both of them.

Grief

For some women I see, especially those who have been trying for a baby for years, the grief can be unbearable, causing them intense pain. Many feel completely disabled and cannot cope with the loss of what, effectively, they never had. Similarly, grief around the loss of a parent, other family member or close friend can also be paralysing. Depending on what the causes are, there are a range of avenues that can be explored. Most of all, women and men struggling with grief need the time and space to be listened to and helped to move on.

Isolation

Many couples I meet with have stopped seeing friends, family and anyone with children. If you have isolated yourself from others, you need support. You need to be helped to realize that communicating with your good friends and family, explaining to them how you are feeling, can only be good for everyone involved. There is no reason for you and your partner to suffer in silence, or alone. You may find, in talking things through, that the people in your life have been through similar trials, and this can be positively liberating and a great source of comfort. These people in your life love you and will without question want to help you in any way they can. Don't cut yourself off from this vital lifeline.

Fear

There are many fears that accompany trying for a baby: Fear that it may never happen, fear that time is running out. I try to help to allay these fears without giving false hope. My advice can take the form of anything from suggesting that a couple move on to IVF to changing clinics, to giving advice about possible treatments if these prove necessary.

If the fears have their root in some kind of earlier trauma or problem, it is, again, important that you try and talk it through with your partner, family, friends and, perhaps, an organized support group or professional counsellor. You owe it to yourself to explore every possible source of help that's available.

Sensual loss

So many women start to feel they are no longer sensual or sexy. They lose their sense of self as a sexual partner. They've been trying for a baby so long, their sexual energy has been diverted away from sex down other paths, in pursuit of a child. Many women in their late thirties say to me they feel old and dried up. They're in a huge panic about their age. Feeling sensual means that you feel young inside. Many women feel, on some level, that their time to get pregnant has past.

The reality is that we fall out of love with ourselves and our bodies. Feeling good about yourself gives you joie de vivre. Hypnosis can help you to see the sensual person within yourself and learn to like and love yourself again.

Mother issues

Very many women that we encounter have had poor relationships with their own mothers, and feel that this in some way is contributing to their problems with conception. Some of you reading this will have dealt with these issues in some other way; for others there may be a hidden impact from negative comments made when they were children, such as 'Don't get pregnant like I did; focus on your career and making money,' 'You were always a difficult child to have around,' 'Don't ever come home pregnant' and 'You don't want children; they only cause you pain and worry.' Such remarks may or may not have been intended spitefully, but they can have long-lasting psychological effects.

In our hypnotherapy work we have frequently come across this sort of 'negative programming', and the depth of its impact may only surface when there appear to be 'unexplained reasons' for a failure to conceive.

Control freaks

Many women are control freaks, regimenting every aspect of their lives. When they can't get pregnant, they can't accept the fact that they cannot control their own bodies. This can have a devastating effect on them. They see having a baby as 'the next natural step', and when it doesn't work for them straight away they are angry and frustrated. They find it difficult to accept that nature will not necessarily be easily controlled. For other women, the lack of control over their bodies that they think pregnancy will bring is too difficult for them to contemplate. On the surface they may appear to want a baby, but subconsciously they are sabotaging their own efforts because they fear losing their financial security or the status and kudos that their career brings them. Some women are the main breadwinners; they control the money, the environment they work in and the relationship. On the surface these women seem very strong, but on the inside, very often, they are incredibly fragile. They need to be able to acknowledge and accept that they don't control everything. Hypnotherapy can help with this.

Abuse

I am always amazed how often past abuse issues come up in consultation. This can have a huge impact on trying for a baby if it has not been dealt with or has been suppressed. Once pregnant, a whole can of worms may be opened. It is also a sensitive issue for women who will be going down an assisted fertility route, who may find that all the scans and probes can be re-traumatizing and bring all sorts of emotions to the surface.

For others, unresolved abuse issues may cause them to harbour a fear that, should they have a child, they may not be able to protect it, as they themselves were once unprotected. They can even come to feel that they don't 'deserve' to have a child. All of this may lead to an inability to conceive.

Secondary fertility problems

There is a large group of women I see who have one or two children already and want another. A lot of them encounter a kind of criticism from others, who try to make them feel guilty or greedy for wanting another child and not being 'content' with what they have. On top of this there is confusion, anger and frustration – 'Why can't I get pregnant now when I've been pregnant with no problems in the past?' They can also feel ashamed about not enjoying the child or children they already have. Often they come to me very confused. Their emotions and feelings are trapped and they don't know how to let go. Age is clearly a big factor here, both in terms of panic that another child will never happen, and also failure to come to terms with the reality of ageing. Some of the women I see carry on in their pursuit to have a baby, to the detriment of everything else in their lives.

Romile, 42, had two children aged 12 and 7. She had been trying for her third child since the second one was three. She had got pregnant once in the ensuing four years, but it had been an ectopic pregnancy and she had lost a Fallopian tube. Romile decided she was not going to go through IVF, as at 42 her chances were not good and her hormone levels not optimum. She had spent the last four years getting different opinions, visiting different doctors and seeking out all sorts of therapists. Her pursuit was all-consuming. She was irritable and snappy with her children and her husband, started to pick fault with everyone, nothing was right. She would wake up in the morning depressed. She couldn't organize her day effectively. Finally, her partner had sat her down and, in tears, told her that he was desperate to make her happy but didn't know how, he couldn't carry on, why couldn't she be happy with what she had? She was constantly pushing him away and he could no longer go on. He wanted the old Romile back. He wanted her to stop and let go.

When she told us all this, we pointed out to her that her relationship was dangerously close to breaking point, that she had a great husband and family, and that her chances of getting pregnant were better naturally but, because she was so consumed with exploring other avenues, she was not having sex often enough. Resentment was building in the relationship and she was pushing her partner away, so of course sex was less likely to occur. We also arranged a session of fertility awareness to help her understand her most fertile time.

We talked a lot about why she felt such a need to have a third child. It turned out that she had never done particularly well or achieved in school, and the one thing she thought she excelled at was being a mother. The thought of her children growing up and not needing her frightened her; she was afraid she'd be left all alone and nobody would need her. We talked about life without another child and used hypnotherapy to help with this. Romile wanted to be able to move on and accept where she was, so that then, if a pregnancy did happen, it would be a bonus.

Depression

Many of the couples I see are depressed, not only about not being able to get pregnant but about their lives being effectively on hold. Some research has been done in this area, but nowhere near enough. In my observation of many couples, depression and stress do contribute to an inability to conceive: the healthy mind/healthy body connection again. Many women are on anti-depressants, which no doubt help in some cases, but also cause reduced libido in some, which defeats the whole object. We therefore look at improving the whole picture, to see what else can be done to improve the situation. We use many typical lifestyle responses to stress and depression: Exercise can boost endorphin levels, as can acupuncture. Meditation, yoga, feeling listened to and having somebody to help you thorough it all – all of these can help with depression and the effects of stress generally.

Relationship Tips

- Take note of your 'predominant' emotion.
- It helps for some clients to write down how they are feeling. Sometimes this may help you to process difficult emotions.
- Both partners need to communicate. Explain how you feel and what the process is like for you.
- Accept one another's opinions and views.
- Accept that you don't have control over your fertility, but you *do* have control over the path you take.
- Make decisions together.
- Don't see your partner as public enemy number one. Remember you are both on the same side. Sometimes men take longer to think things through and get to the same level as their partners.
- You are both changing. Tell each other what you have learned as you go along. This is particularly useful if you have had a failed IVF attempt. Work out strategies to support each other emotionally.

How Hypnotherapy Can Help

Hypnotherapy has had a bad press for a long time, but has now gained the respect of the medical establishment and is recognized as a very useful tool in helping reduce stress levels and aid relaxation. It has also been seen to have some success with cases of unexplained infertility – where no physical cause has been found on investigation. My feeling is that if you try to separate the emotional from the physical, when it comes to fertility, you will fail to help couples. In particular, women who have had a termination or suffered a miscarriage, violence or abuse can be helped to release the stress of the trauma and grief, and let go of the past, through hypnotherapy.

A qualified and experienced hypnotherapist works with a fully conscious person, helping them reach a profound state of relaxation where the subconscious part of the brain is accessed and positive suggestions can be made that release deep-seated fears and phobias. It is completely safe and very effective.

In addition to dealing with deep-seated fears, hypnotherapy is effective in stress-reduction, and this in turn allows for hormonal rebalancing. This has been seen in cases where there is too much prolactin being produced, which can inhibit ovulation.

Most people are receptive to hypnotherapy, and it can only work with a person's consent. Hypnosis evokes a comfortable and relaxed state of being which you can then re-create on your own – in fact, one of the many benefits of hypnotherapy is that, once introduced to the technique, it's possible to learn how to create a relaxed and meditative state at will, for yourself. If taught this technique, it can be combined with visualization and affirmations to create a relaxed and receptive state of mind.

Maureen Kiely, our Clinical Hypnotherapist, says, 'Many of the clients I see have had their confidence shattered by the inability to conceive or maintain a pregnancy to full term. My role is to help build their belief in the possibility of pregnancy and giving birth. For many clients there are unexplained issues which contribute to this sense of failure or disbelief in themselves. Some of these issues or blocks may be hampering fertility and conception.'

Hypnotherapy can help by enabling clients to understand the nature of their emotional block, acknowledge its effect and change its impact in order to let go and move on.

Hypnotherapy allows fears to be expressed in a safe way, and helps men and women to gain a realistic assessment of their needs and desires. This allows for an honest appraisal of the situation and provides strategies for building self-confidence. We work with controlling those areas that can be controlled (such as emotional responses), and helping women and men to accept that they do not control the universe; they have to work with what they have. What you can control is your positivity!

One of our clients, for example, was having trouble with 'perform-ance anxiety' and expressed his wish for help in this area. Though deeply sceptical, declaring his 'total disbelief in anything like hyp-notherapy actually working,' he had the good grace to try it – and then to apologize when he reported, after one session of hypnotherapy: 'It was incredible; I did not believe it was possible but, yes, everything is back in working order and we are full steam ahead.'

By dealing with the underlying emotional issues and increasing his libido response he was more able to understand the reasons why he was failing to maintain an erection, and this helped him to develop strategies to regain his performance and lose the anxiety!

Low self-esteem is another problem that hypnotherapy can address. Feelings of low self-esteem can come from anywhere – childhood, poor body image, negative relationships – and of course if you have been trying for a baby for a while, it can be all too easy to start to feel bad about yourself. What hypnotherapy can do here is build and develop feelings of self-worth, so you get some of your confidence back.

When it comes to countering the effects of negative messages a man or woman may have been exposed to in childhood, hypnosis can help to replace these negative messages with beneficial, nurturing and motivating ones that will encourage emotional and psychological well-being. This in turn leads to increased self-esteem and self-worth, and encourages confidence. When you believe something is possible and achievable, you are on the right road to pregnancy and parenthood.

For the control freaks among us, hypnotherapy can help you to relax and let go, helping you to dissociate from the situation and providing you with strategies for 'drifting to a safe place'.

For some women who have been abused, their own 'inner child' remains abused and hurt. Through careful work with hypnosis we can ameliorate the harm and provide a more adult response to deal with the emotional scarring and psychological damage that can result in a woman not embracing her own womanhood.

The inner child is the innocent, defenceless child you once were. Imagine a child who is beaten or bullied every time she falls short of whatever task or behaviour the adults around her require. Sooner or later that child's confidence and spirit will be broken and she will go through life with a distorted view of the world and herself. The work we do with a person's inner child can be very powerful in helping women to be kind to their inner child and not beat themselves up. Instead, we help them learn to be supportive of and encouraging to their inner child. This, in turn, reminds women of their own spontaneity and joie de vivre. Life can be full and does not have to be a trial – many times women have lost their capacity to see the fun in life. Hypnotherapy and work on the inner child helps them to reclaim this valuable inner gift.

Creative Visualization

Hypnotherapy is also very useful in enabling clients to visualize and create positive outcomes – from being able to see themselves pregnant to being able to visualize embryos embedding while undergoing egg harvesting or implantation in IVF. Much of our recent work has also included the use of visualization to dampen down overactive natural killer cells by harnessing the unconscious to affect the immune system. This is achieved through trance work, which operates specifically on a 'brain as a control-room' concept which has been used successfully with patients with cancer in clinical settings, who have increased their own natural healing abilities and natural killer cells to stimulate enhanced immune responses. We reverse this concept for our work in fertility.

Visualization can also be used to help a woman to see herself with a baby, to be able to see the embryo into the endometrium. Some women panic, thinking they won't be able to visualize this properly. We work with them to help them form their own unique imagery.

One way we do this is with the 'fertile garden' exercise. We have many laughs with clients who worry they are over-watering their gardens or there are too many weeds.

Many women worry that they won't visualize properly. Let me assure you that this is a very simple process, takes around five minutes to learn, gives you a real sense of calm and tranquillity and also helps you to become proactive in whatever process you are going through.

The following visualization exercise may be used as a basic 'recipe' – all you have to add is your unique circumstances or desired result. So you can use this technique whether you are trying to reduce your FSH levels, visualize a good egg harvest or imagine yourself in full, healthy pregnancy.

We encourage women to visualize at every stage of their personal journey, be it IVF or natural conception. If you feel you are not particularly good at imagining or visualizing, try looking on the Internet for pictures or use the diagram on page 84 to help. You can even use an image of a colour or symbol to represent what you want to visualize. For some people, an aroma or sound may stimulate a memory and help them to focus. One woman I worked with could not picture anything but was able to recall the smell of baby lotion, which reminded her of babies! We are all unique individuals, so you need to do what is right for you and to work with what works for you!

In Chinese medicine, wherever you visualize in your body, your *qi* follows.

1. Find a quiet spot where you will be undisturbed. This should be a spot where you feel safe, unselfconscious, warm and cozy.

2. Unplug the telephone, turn off your mobile. Inform people who may want to contact you that you will be unavailable for this period of time. You will need around 20 minutes.

3. Support your back on a bed in a semi-seated position – legs up is the best position.

4. Place your hands on your lower abdomen.

5. The breath and breathing are very important. We are aiming for abdominal breathing. We tend to breathe very shallowly; we need to create a greater exchange of oxygen flowing through the body to gain a good relaxation response.

6. Begin by breathing normally, then take a deep, slow breath, through your nose. Notice how your abdomen starts to expand – then exhale through your mouth. Breathe in a way that is comfortable for you.

7. Continue breathing for 5 minutes in this slower, more conscious way.

8. Remain focused, letting any unnecessary thoughts just drift away. Don't bother to fight them, just allow them to emerge and then see them travel away out of focus.

9. Focus on the top of your head and allow the relaxation to flow down through your head to your forehead.

10. Allow the relaxation to continue to flow down to your cheekbones and jawbone.

11. Allow the relaxation to flow to your neck, shoulders and down through your arms to your hands.

12. Allow the relaxation to flow down through your chest and stomach, warming your abdomen on the way.

13. Allow the relaxation to flow down through your pelvic region. Feel it grow soft and warm.

14. Allow the relaxation to flow down through your upper legs, down through your lower legs and all the way down to your feet and toes.

15. Now picture your favourite place to relax. Gently float and drift to this place.

16. Now, feeling relaxed, safe and secure – begin to visualize.

Here are some hints from our Clinical Hypnotherapist, Maureen Kiely, to help you get started:

• Imagine the mind has a control room marked Fertility and Reproduction. You have the key. Go into the room and see the controls for your FSH. Imagine a dial and turn down the levels. Use this for any levels you wish to control. You can return and check to make any further adjustments as and when required.

• When you are waiting after your embryos have been implanted, imagine a good, healthy environment for them – picture a rich, vibrant red cushion with 'Welcome' written on it. Imagine the embryos burrowing and nestling in, warm, safe and secure. Imagine them being protected and guarded by your vigilant subconscious mind.

- Picture yourself in a tranquil, safe environment, like a garden on a warm summer's day, pushing a pram back and forth, feeling the weight of the baby in the pram and maybe singing the baby to sleep.

Give your imagination free rein here. Allow yourself to be creative, free, unselfconscious and prepared to follow your heart's wishes.

Finding the Right Therapist

If you are going to have hypnosis, it is crucial to the success of the treatment that you choose a therapist who has been recommended to you. Never let anybody impose their views on you; build up a rapport with the therapist. If you don't have this, find another therapist. You need to be able to feel safe about disclosing information and opening up. Generally you should feel good and positive after a session. Some sessions may be tearful, but a skilled therapist will be able to deal with this in a supportive and sympathetic way.

Apart from hypnosis, there are other therapies that can help you to deal with your emotions, such as counselling or cognitive therapy.

traditional chinese medicine

Ancient versus Modern

The ancient Chinese followed the laws of nature. They had a set of rules which are just as relevant to our health today as they were thousands of years ago.

Ancient Chinese practitioners did not have the blood tests and scans we have today; they would make a diagnosis and prescribe treatments based on observation alone. The colour or hue around a patient's eyes, the sound of his or her voice and the odour and emotions the person displayed – all of these would be used when making a diagnosis, and all involved close study of the patient. Sadly, in spite of all of today's wonderful technology doctors are getting further and further away from truly being *with* their patients. Medicine is preoccupied with putting information about a patient straight into a computer, filling in forms and generally missing out on what is going on with the patient sitting right there in the room. Chinese medicine describes processes inside and outside the body in energetic terms. Western medicine describes these same processes in physiological and biochemical ways.

I have to say that this is also happening in other forms of complementary medicine, where new-age machines, hair analyses and fancy tests are more and more replacing being *with* the patient and meeting his or her emotional needs. I learn so much about a client by just being there, and much of my work is spent listening to and truly connecting with individuals or a couple.

Yin and Yang

The ancient Chinese looked at nature as it exists in each and every one of us. They were very tuned in to the changing seasons and cycles. They believed that the body's *qi*, or life-force, is influenced by two opposing forces: yin and yang. These are co-dependent – existing side by side – and have to be in balance for the body to work most effectively.

Yin is equated with the dark, with stillness, quiet, winter and the cold. The Yin of a person is the ability to be calm, quiet and still, and to sleep.

Yang is warm, day, active and hot. The Yang of a person is the ability to communicate, work and be active.

As I've mentioned elsewhere in this book, so many of the couples I see have lost the balance in their lives, most often with too much Yang and not enough Yin!

Qi

According to the beliefs of Traditional Chinese Medicine (TCM), we all have a vital life-force, *qi*, which moves along invisible pathways in the body called *meridians*. The meridians are named for the major organs through which they pass, such as the lung, spleen, heart, kidney, liver, bladder, stomach and large intestine meridians, and there are also meridians with their own unique names: the conception vessel (running right through the midline of the body and considered a very important meridian for fertility), and the governing vessel (which runs up through the spine).

Along each meridian are recognized acupuncture points (for more about acupuncture, see below, page 219). It is these points that are used by an acupuncturist to restore the flow of *qi*, strengthen the relevant organ and to restore balance.

Although the concept of *qi* has always met with scepticism and resistance from Western medicine, we all talk about our energy levels every day. Energy is the life-force that is in every cell of our bodies.

In TCM it is believed that there are 365 acupoints located along the meridians; these are like tiny valves along which the flow of *qi* can be regulated. Some acupuncture points are named for their (well-researched) relevance to certain bodily processes. The Chinese have some wonderful names for the acupoints that are particularly relevant for fertility: Palace of the Child, Gate of Life, Sea of Qi, Door of Infants, and Palace of Weariness. Many of these points lie along the lower abdomen.

Qi flows through the meridian system. If your body is in balance, you will not be aware of anything. Any pain or discomfort, however, will indicate a blockage in the flow of *qi*. The flow of *qi* is affected by external factors such as cold, damp, heat and wind, and internal ones such as worry, anger, fear and grief. As long as the *qi* is flowing smoothly through the meridians, body systems function well. Many of us, however, have a constitutional weakness in one organ or another, and if the energy from one organ is weak, this puts the whole body out of balance. Energetically, in Chinese medicine each emotion is linked to an organ: the stomach, for example, is associated with worry. The liver is associated with anger and is important in Chinese medicine for ovulation. PMT is believed to be an outcome of liver stagnation.

The Kidneys

The kidneys have a particular significance in Chinese medicine: They govern reproduction, they are important for bones, teeth, marrow and brain function. According to TCM, many women who are having trouble conceiving or carrying a baby have weak kidney energy. This is because the kidneys are believed to store reproductive *jing. Jing* is our essence. Strong *jing* results in strong sperm in men, strong eggs in women and strong and healthy children.

The kidneys provide essence or *jing* for the uterus, and declining kidney energy equates in Western medicine to declining hormone levels as a woman gets older. Also, in TCM the kidneys are considered important for our genetic material.

After a TCM diagnosis, many women are found to have a weakness in their kidney energy. The (very common) symptoms of this include:

- low backache around period times
- scanty cervical mucus
- low libido
- night sweats
- fearfulness.

Acupuncture along certain points of the kidney meridian builds up kidney energy.

In TCM, fear is the emotion associated with the kidneys. When you think about it, the adrenal glands sit on top of the kidneys, and adrenal stress stimulates our bodies into fight or flight mode. In Chinese medicine, fear is believe to cause the *qi* to sink, and sinking *qi* is associated with fertility problems. Kidney *jing* can also get 'used up' as a result of menstruation, stress, pregnancy or miscarriage.

Treatment to restore kidney balance and energy, which may have become depleted through repeated miscarriages or IVF treatment, can be very effective. Acupuncture can be used to focus on the meridians that help build up kidney *jing*. Alongside this, lifestyle advice is given on how to boost the kidney energy: cutting out stimulants that put stress on the adrenals, eating the right foods, meditating, using relaxation techniques, getting enough sleep and, particularly, the importance of resting each day between 5 and 7 p.m. (the time of day associated, in TCM, with kidney energy – see page 222).

In TCM it is believed that we inherit our kidney *jing* from our parents. Kidney *jing* play a vital role in all stages of a woman's life, from puberty and her fertile years through to the menopause. It also affects her libido. In terms of Western medicine, kidney *jing* equates to the ovaries and pituitary gland.

The Blood

In Western medicine the blood is seen as a collection of cells that circulates through the body, nourishing, maintaining and oxygenating the system. Chinese medicine considers the blood as housing our spirit. This may sound a bit strange, but we can easily equate this with Western medicine's ideas about conditions such as anaemia, which is called 'blood deficiency' in Chinese medicine. Very often when a woman is anaemic, she is pale, exhausted, breathless, dizzy and low in spirits, and usually very tearful. In Chinese medicine, acupuncture is used to build the blood – research has shown that certain points such as stomach 36 increase the haemoglobin in the blood. Foods will also be suggested that can help to build the blood.

Everything about a woman's menstrual blood flow is significant in knowing which points to use and which patterns you are looking for. For example, blood stagnation (when the blood is not moving efficiently through the body) is seen, in TCM, to be the cause of menstrual clots, fibroids and endometriosis.

In Chinese medicine, the blood has a special relationship with three organs: the heart, the liver and the spleen. In Chinese medicine the heart is the seat of our emotions, and supplies blood for the uterus and the conception vessel. The acupuncture points that connect the heart and uterus are considered very important for fertility. Very often if the heart is upset or broken, it is believed that the spirit will be weak.

Menstrual Cycles

Women have lost an awareness of their menstrual cycles. In Chinese medicine, questioning a woman about her menstrual cycle can be crucial when it comes to prescribing the right treatment. I am amazed that women rely on painkillers so much for period pain – if everything is working normally there should not be a lot of pain during your cycle.

Acupuncture can certainly help with painful periods. Suggested lifestyle factors to augment the benefits of acupuncture would include:

- Avoiding the use of tampons, if at all possible.
- No exercise during a period – you need to build up your energy, not deplete it.
- No swimming during a period, as this makes the lower area of the body very cold.
- No sex during a period – many cultures across the world follow this maxim, and recognize that many women feel very tired during this stage and that this is a time for reflection.

My Experience of Acupuncture

My introduction to acupuncture came following the birth of my son. At the time I was working as a community midwife, my pregnancy had been particularly difficult, I was sick and had lost a lot of weight. After the birth the weight continued to drop off, I was physically exhausted and emotionally fragile and flat. This, plus lack of sleep, meant I had no appreciation or enjoyment for anything. My GP was great, but his only solution was to give me anti-depressants.

Then a friend suggested I try acupuncture. Up until that point I thought it was just for aches and pains; I had no idea how it might help with post-natal depression.

The practitioner I saw was a Five-Element practitioner (see page 223). He diagnosed my element as Fire. Basically, he said my fire had 'gone out'. I was, as anyone could recognize, 'burnt out'.

I went for six sessions of acupuncture and started taking a real interest in my own health, reading up about nutrition and diet. When I started to learn about acupuncture I was fascinated by how much common sense was behind it. The philosophy that underlies acupuncture is all about balance and harmony, and staying within the laws of nature (the seasons, for example) to keep healthy. Today we have lost touch with so much of this ancient wisdom. We have forgotten our own innate knowledge that winter is a time to build up our reserves, a time when the evenings draw in early and we are meant to go to bed earlier and get plenty of sleep to recharge our batteries. (This is why, in other parts of this book, the focus is on eating warming foods to combat the cold and boost your fertility, and on measures to keep yourself warm – particularly your feet, abdomen and lower back – especially during your period.) As for spring, this is the time when your own inner 'sap' starts to rise. You feel more like being outside and socializing in the evenings. Most of us also intuitively feel the urge to 'spring-clean' – and this can include detoxing (our own, internal spring-clean). In summer, socializing hits its peak as the daylight lasts for most of the day. In autumn, we can again begin to feel the need to stock up (bring in the harvest) and prepare for the dark winter days ahead.

Assessment and Diagnosis

By talking with a couple who have come to see me, and through detailed questions and observations, I pick up patterns of disharmony in the meridian system – and then use acupuncture points to correct them. Acupuncture is particularly useful for helping couples to conceive, not least because it very effectively treats the problems that can reduce fertility.

When I see a couple, I base my assessment of where they are at by using my experience as an acupuncturist and my knowledge of the Five Elements (see page 223) and of the many other tenets of Traditional Chinese Medicine.

My main aim is to be with the couple and do my very best to understand what is going on with them, their story so far.

The way they walk into the room, how they hold themselves, how they sit, their body language and the dynamic between them – I observe all of these carefully and they are all very important to my diagnosis. Using the ideas behind Five Element diagnosis, I am interested in the sound of their voices, their predominant emotion (grief, fear, worry, anger) and the colour of different areas of their faces. Just being with them, listening to what they are saying (or not saying), really paying attention to how they are communicating is so important in seeing where any constitutional weaknesses are, in understanding where they are coming from and in meeting their emotional needs.

In terms of the teachings of TCM, this part of making a diagnosis also involves asking specific questions about their body systems, the woman's periods, blood flow and colour of the blood, whether she ever has any clots, etc.

The Tongue

After these questions I will ask the woman to lie down and I will examine her tongue. In TCM, the different areas of the tongue have a great deal to tell us about a person's state of physical and emotional health because they relate to different areas of the body. It's not that long ago that even Western doctors would examine the tongue to make a diagnosis. In TCM we look for the colour, coating, any cracks – these reveal weaknesses elsewhere in the body. The tongue's coating tells us about a person's constitution: is she constitutionally hot or cold?

The Abdomen

Next I will feel a woman's lower abdomen (this is called 'abdominal palpation') to see if it is warm or not. If it is cold, I will use acupuncture needles at certain acupoints to infuse the point with deep heat using a herb called *moxa*.

Palpating the abdomen is also important for locating any areas of tension or tenderness, which can be treated with massage to relax and ease them. (For more about this, see page 229.)

The 24-hour clock

Understanding our 24-hour clock is an important diagnostic tool. Each meridian has a peak two-hour period during the day, and a time for resting. This is helpful in diagnosis. If there are any problems with pain or sleep, for example, you find out what time of day this is a problem for the client – this helps build a picture of that person. It is also helpful as part of lifestyle advice given to clients. The peak time for the stomach is 7 to 9 a.m., for example, so this is when you should eat a good breakfast. Likewise the 'rest time' for the stomach is 7 to 9 p.m., and so you shouldn't eat during this time at all – yet most of us are in the habit of eating at precisely this time!

Peak Times

7–9 a.m.	Stomach
9–11 a.m.	Spleen
11–1 p.m.	Heart
1–3 p.m.	Small intestine
3–5 p.m.	Bladder
5–7 p.m.	Kidney
7–9 p.m.	Pericardium
9–11 p.m.	Circulation and sex organs
11 p.m.–1 a.m.	Gall bladder
1–3 a.m.	Liver
3–5 a.m.	Lung
5–7 a.m.	Colon

PULSES

Chinese medicine focuses on six pulses on each hand. These are superficial or deep – practitioners are checking for the *quality* of each pulse, not just its speed. With women, these pulses vary throughout a menstrual cycle, and so provide a crucial aid to diagnosis.

I also look at body temperature, particularly of the abdomen in women. The temperature of the abdomen should be even all over, because in Traditional Chinese Medicine it's not considered possible to nourish a baby in a 'cold' abdomen. I have noticed that many of my female clients who are having trouble conceiving have a lower abdomen that is cold to the touch. I try to get my clients to use a hot water bottle in the evenings to bring heat to this part of the body during the first half of their cycle.

A Five Element Diagnosis

TCM works in harmony with nature's seasons and cycles. The ancient Chinese made a correlation between the seasons and the five elements: fire, wood, earth, water and metal. Early masters recognized that these elements were within us as well as all around us.

According to the teachings of TCM, the Five Elements are also related to the five vital organs of the body – the heart, kidneys, liver, lungs and spleen. So, for example, the liver is related to wood and to spring. Each of us is a combination of all five elements, but we tend to have a dominant element which helps to define us. Creating a balance of the elements is part of achieving positive health. This is the way I diagnose clients, and it helps me to meet their emotional needs and gain a much greater understanding of them as individuals.

Some of you reading this maybe wondering what Five Element acupuncture has got to do with helping you get pregnant. Each person I see comes with a unique package of her own, and presents with a predominant emotion. Look around at people you know: some are always laughing and happy, some whinge non-stop, some like to have a moan occasionally, some are fearful, some very kind and caring, some sympathetic, some always seem angry.

Within the Five Element framework in which I trained, emotional engagement and rapport with the client are paramount to the healing process. I have to be able to experience and feel within me the emotions that my patient is feeling; I have to be able to connect with them. To make a diagnosis I assess what particular element the patient is. I look at the colour of her face, the sound of her voice, her unique scent and the emotions she displays (joy or the lack of it, anger, fear, worry, grief). Once I can pinpoint their primary Element I am able to see certain patterns emerging that are linked to certain organs. The ancient Chinese believed that emotions affect organs and energy flow. In Western medicine no such link is made. For the Chinese, anger knots the liver *qi* and is related to PMS, etc., worry affects the stomach. I always ask where a person feels an emotion – the chest, the stomach, neck, abdomen, gut, etc. – we all have our weak spots. The use of certain acupuncture points can treat each area.

Orthodox medicine compartmentalizes us; TCM sees all parts as constituents of the whole. As part of my diagnosis, I always used TCM and the Five Elements as a constitutional approach. If you can find a practitioner near you, please do give it a try – many women swear by its positive effects on fertility.

I am indebted to Gerad Kite, master in Five Element acupuncture, for his contribution to the following explanation of this comprehensive system.

> *The ancient Chinese were concerned with all that was 'real', and although they were great thinkers and scholars, unbelievably advanced for their time, all of Chinese thought was based on actual human experience rather than conjecture. They looked at the sky above them and contemplated the universe, they looked at the people around them and experienced humanity, and they looked deep within themselves and discovered the 'self'. They instinctively understood that everything in manifestation came from the same origin. Most*

importantly, they used their senses to harvest this information to develop their wisdom, as what we as humans see, hear, smell and feel is our only truth.

When we are born, our power of thought is barely developed – so we start to collect information about ourselves, the people around us and our environment through our senses. We look around at the strange shapes and movements, we hear different noises – some mechanical, some human – we begin to experience ourselves through the development of our emotions.

The ancient Chinese worked with natural laws to maintain good health. They looked at the whole and then conceptually broke it down into Five Phases or Elements in order to understand the perfect whole. A Five Element diagnosis, then, is a key to really understanding and being able to meet the emotional needs of a patient.

The easiest way to understand the Five Elements is to look at the natural cycle of the seasons. Our experience of any particular year is never exactly the same, but we are aware of a cycle that repeats itself continuously, winter followed by spring, summer by late summer and autumn. This cycle creates the year, just as the Five Elements create us.

The greatest skill of an acupuncturist is the ability to *be* with a patient in the way the patient needs. We need to be able to sense what each individual needs to get better, not just in the placing of our needles but more importantly in how we *are* and how we communicate with the patient.

It can be very interesting, great fun and sometimes very illuminating to discover your own particular element, though of course it's best to leave a proper diagnosis to a practitioner. So take a look at the following descriptions, but keep in mind that making your own, subjective diagnosis is difficult.

Water (Blue/Groaning/Putrefaction/ Fear/Kidneys and Bladder/Winter)

Water types can be very driven, ambitious and wilful, feeling compelled to move relentlessly towards fulfilling their potential. Conversely they can feel impotent, having no power to exert their will in the world, not knowing who they are or what they want.

The emotion of Water is fear. Fear affects the adrenal glands.

The season associated with Water is winter, a time when we should be building up our reserves.

Fire (Red/Laughter/Scorching/Joy/ Heart and Circulation/Summer)

Fire types are very 'up and down' emotionally. They can be great fun and a real laugh, while also being very sensitive and vulnerable. They are very conscious of how they are seen by others, and other points of view are very important to them. The real challenge of Fire types is moderation, as they tend to swing from one extreme to another in everything that they do. The challenge for Fire types is to learn just to be and to relax. At the opposite extreme, some Fire types can be completely lacking in joy – true Victor Meldrew types who cannot raise a spark. Fire types need warmth and touch.

Wood (Green/Shouting/Rancidity/ Anger/Liver and Gallbladder/Spring)

Wood types love to plan, to move forward. They are very challenging and do not suffer fools gladly. They need a worthy opponent. Habitually they respond with anger, a natural emotion within them regardless of the situation – yet they do not see themselves as angry. They want and need to grow. Wood types can be aggressive but at the opposite extreme can be very meek, timid and unassertive.

Metal (White/Weeping/Rot/Grief/ Lungs and Colon/Autumn)

In balance, Metal types are brilliant and awe-inspiring to those around them. They make all the connections and are firing on all cylinders. If *qi* is out of balance, however, Metal types become completely disconnected with the world and the people around them. They hold on to every negative thought and find it hard to let go; they bear grudges and become critical and negative. Others can find their grief difficult to be around. Emotionally it's important to help Metal-types learn to reconnect so that they can work things out for themselves.

The season associated with Metal is autumn.

Earth (Yellow/Singing/Fragrance/ Sympathy/Stomach and Spleen/Late Summer)

Earth types are highly sensitive, care deeply about the needs of others and are eager to please. When *qi* is balanced, they are very sympathetic and lovely to be around. If *qi* is out of balance, however, their perspective can get distorted and they start to feel like a victim. This can become a burden for and a drain on others. Earth types are often real worriers, going round and round in circles trying to sort things out.

The time of year associated with the Earth element is late summer.

Five Element acupuncture is so much a part of my practice, and so helpful when it comes to helping clients achieve pregnancy, that it informs my very first impressions of clients as I meet them. I find it extremely helpful in making a first assessment, and also in devising a focus for the assistance and treatment a couple might need.

Treatment

When it comes to fertility, the mind/body link is integral to the way a couple – and women in particular – approach pregnancy. This is because the hormonal component of a woman's fertility is so closely related to her sense of emotional well-being. Because of this, when there are difficulties in conceiving, it is more important than ever to take a holistic approach.

As a practising and experienced midwife, I have extended my clinical practice to incorporate what couples need emotionally, and this is the strength of Five Element acupuncture, which doesn't separate the mind, body and spirit, but regards them as all parts of the same whole.

There is a growing body of research evidence which shows that acupuncture can help:

- correct irregular cycles
- boost ovulation
- balance hormones
- improve pelvic blood flow
- increase the endometrial lining
- reduce stress by releasing endorphins
- improve sperm counts
- boost the immune system.

Auricular (Ear) Acupuncture

A lot of research has also been done on the use of auricular acupuncture, where the meridians in the ear are used for treatment. In Traditional Chinese Medicine the ear is likened to an inverted foetus. All the major meridians cross the ear, which has 120 acupoints. Just as, in reflexology, points along the feet are seen to correspond with organs and systems elsewhere in the body, in Chinese medicine the ear is thought to be significant for its many useful acupoints. Ear acupuncture has been used for fertility treatment and is common in clinics to help with drug addiction and giving up smoking. In the case of fertility, it is of particular value when treating hormonal imbalances. There is plenty of research to show how ear acupuncture can improve fertility.

Scars

Scars are very important in Chinese medicine. Following surgery, the body usually heals itself – however, for some women it doesn't and the area around the scar can remain very cold.

Abdominal Massage

I first experienced abdominal massage when I was in Thailand; I now incorporate it in my practice. It originated with Taoist monks, who used it to help detoxify and strengthen the lower abdomen. It is particularly useful for relaxing tension in the abdomen and promoting blood flow.

So many of the women I see have very tense lower abdomens. I start off an abdominal massage by pressing key acupoints around the navel, checking for tenderness. I then begin a gentle massage using four fingers of my hand in a circular movement around the navel, spreading out to the whole of the abdomen. In this way I can take note of any discomfort, any tension or knots in the abdomen. This massage improves the blood flow, detoxifying the systems by working on the lymph nodes directly underneath.

Electro-acupuncture

Electro-acupuncture involves inserting acupuncture needles into acu-points and then passing a low-frequency electrical current via small clips attached to the needles. I often use electro-acupuncture when treating clients, as this boosts the treatment's effectiveness. It also has the capacity to relieve pain, boost ovulation, help with endorphin release and regulate a woman's fertility cycle. A Swedish study carried out in 1996 found that electro-acupuncture improved the blood flow to the womb in women with fertility problems. A good blood supply ensures adequate nourishment for an embryo, and also that the womb is warm – both very important for conception. What happens naturally in the body is that the hormone progesterone helps the body tempera-ture to rise in readiness for a growing embryo. The conception vessel runs through the abdomen, and many important acupuncture points for fertility lie here. I usually use needles with *moxa* on them, which puts a nice deep heat down the needle and along the abdomen in the first half of the cycle. I also usually encourage clients to use a hot water bot-tle or heating pad for 5 or 10 minutes in the evening to heat up the lower abdomen. Heat acts as vasodilator, which means it opens up the blood vessels and improves the blood supply. Research has also shown that acupuncture improves pelvic blood supply – and when current fashion trends mean that this part of the body is exposed more often than not, making sure it gets some warmth is particularly important!

In Chinese medicine we also use yang foods to help women trying for a baby. These are warming foods that help to keep the *qi* flowing. Too many cold and raw foods stagnate the *qi*.

Treatment Protocols

I have different protocols that I use depending on the client. Generally clients will have weekly treatments for four to six weeks, then spread out to monthly maintenance treatments. During assisted fertility we usually do a treatment prior to the start and then treat two to three times a week during stimulation and between egg collection and transfer, and then 10 days after transfer.

Research

Acupuncture has been shown to:
- lower excess levels of FSH (follicle-stimulating hormone)
- regulate the menstrual cycle – in particular shortening long cycles
- relieve symptoms of endometriosis
- induce ovulation in women with PCOS (polycystic ovary syndrome)
- improve the concentration and motility of sperm
- release endorphins
- improve general health.

Acupuncture can be very beneficial for improving sperm counts. Energetically the testes are directly linked to the kidneys, so acupuncture treatment would be along the kidney meridian. Acupuncture has also been used successfully to increase sperm motility.

Remember, it is important when you choose a therapy or therapist that you feel happy with the treatment that you are getting. Try and get several word-of-mouth recommendations. Support groups can be useful for this. Phone around and chat to the therapists to find out their experience of treating women trying to get pregnant. Be wary of false hopes or promises; trust your instincts and limit the time you spend on a particular therapy to a couple of months. Keep checking for improvements and changes all along the way.

While research shows that acupuncture can boost endorphin levels, improve blood flow and help regulate the body's cycles and hormone levels, I think its success has as much to do with the practitioner's individual approach. Truly *being* with a patient is what makes all the difference. To me there is nothing esoteric or mystical about acupuncture, it's just a simple and direct approach to understanding life and nature.

I don't recommend the use of acupuncture in isolation when it comes to promoting fertility. Although highly effective, acupuncture has little value if nutrition is poor, or the body is dealing with lifestyle factors that drain its resources. The body will always get what it needs to survive, until the demand is too great and illness occurs, and in these cases fertility demands will come a poor second. It is imperative, if conception and pregnancy is the goal, to take a holistic view of treatment, of which acupuncture can play an invaluable role, and be prepared to participate actively in making the lifestyle and nutritional changes that are necessary.

part three
fertility problems and solutions

fertility work-up

When There Are Problems Conceiving

However many steps you take to ensure you and your partner are in the best possible physical and emotional health for conception, there are inevitably going to be problems for some couples. Some of these problems can be relatively easy to overcome, but for others medical intervention may be the only option.

For many couples, the spectre of infertility is never far from their minds, whether or not there is a logical reason why this might be true for them. It's important, therefore, to remember what the definitions are, and to understand that infertility isn't necessarily a finite diagnosis, but may be just a transitory problem. It is equally important to remember that, without a full work-up to find the possible cause, assisted conception is not always the next step. And even if it comes to this, in the end, then there is a great deal that a couple can do to help ensure a positive outcome (see page 311).

Some couples are aware – perhaps because of the woman's irregular cycle – that there may be problems. For others there may be a general health problem, but not one they thought might be related to getting pregnant. For still others there may be a completely hidden problem which neither partner is aware of. One of the reasons our clinic offers couples very detailed questionnaires is to provide us with an immediate overview of some of the problems that can arise and – with treatment – be overcome.

It is my recommendation that every couple considering pregnancy should have a basic fertility check (see page xv) which covers age, weight, general health, menstrual and contraceptive history, family history, sexual history, previous illnesses and operations, for example. This chapter will take a close look at the factors that can affect your fertility, the investigations used to pinpoint a problem and some of the ways you can help yourself. The first half explores factors affecting women's fertility; while the latter part looks at men's fertility in detail.

On average, 1 in 7 couples in the UK will seek medical advice over difficulties in getting pregnant, though a couple is not regarded as 'infertile' until they have failed to conceive after 12 months of unprotected intercourse.

Doctors generally advise that you seek their help about problems conceiving if:

- you are a woman aged between 30 and 35 and have been having unprotected intercourse for a year
- you are a woman aged 35 and have been having unprotected intercourse for six months.

Some experts recommend that if you have learned about fertility awareness and you have been having lots of sex targeted to your most fertile time, then it is reasonable to consider initial tests (such as hormone tests) earlier – such as after six months of 'targeted' sex regardless of your age.

The three primary reasons for a failure to conceive are:

1. eggs not being released
2. eggs not passing down into the Fallopian tubes
3. sperm problems.

These three reasons will be related to:

- hormonal problems
- tubal problems
- structural problems
- medical problems (e.g. endometriosis)

or may remain unexplained.

Factors Affecting Fertility

While around 15 per cent of all couples of reproductive age will have a fertility problem of some sort, this will of course be influenced by a number of factors:

- age
- contraceptive history
- sexual history
- menstrual cycle
- lifestyle factors
- underlying medical disorders
- underlying reproductive disorders
- immune system problems.

Let's take a look at each of these in turn.

Age

Inevitably, it is the age of the woman that most closely influences whether there is a problem; male fertility does decline with age, but not as dramatically. In every case, however, the benefits of general good health in both partners can make a big difference.

A woman has a 25 per cent chance of conceiving per cycle, as long as there are no health problems, ovulation occurs and she is having unprotected intercourse at her most fertile time.

Given this, it's important to know when to seek help. An initial step is to have a full assessment. I advise any couple who are planning a pregnancy to do this, because having a baseline before you start can be very useful if there are problems later on – it shortens the process of investigations which can arise and, if you are over 35, this can make all the difference to the outcome.

Contraceptive History

Factors like how long you have been on the Pill, if you have had an IUD or used depo-prevera (given as an injection that lasts for three months) or a contraceptive implant will all need to be considered if a couple are having problems conceiving, as having used any of these can delay conception.

Sexual History

I get many of the couples I see to have a full sexual health screen before they start trying for a baby, and particularly if they have never been checked before. In some cases this can be done at their local clinic or hospital (many hospitals have units attached where you can have tests carried out), although it can be difficult to get a full screen on the NHS and it may have to be done privately. (This is discussed in more detail in the Lifestyle chapter.)

A man's or woman's fertility can easily be affected by an infection in the reproductive organs. This may be something as simple and easily treated as thrush, or something as damaging as chlamydia, which can lead to pelvic inflammatory disease (PID) and blocked tubes. In men, an infection can cause blocked ducts in the testes, prostate problems and/or damaged sperm. In women, not only can the Fallopian tubes be blocked (with the attendant risk of an ectopic pregnancy), but the risk of early miscarriage is also increased. One problem of infections like chlamydia is that approximately 70–80 per cent of women sufferers can experience no symptoms at all, so they may pass it on unwittingly or suffer internal damage before they even know they have it. Sexually transmitted infections (STIs) are on the increase, and every new relationship or change of partners in your past could have left you with an underlying or dormant condition you may not even be aware of. For couples trying to conceive, and therefore (of course) not using condoms, any existing infection will easily be passed between partners.

I encourage couples to see fertility infection screening as a positive, not a negative. If infections are found, they can be either treated or monitored – in my experience the improvements to fertility after treatment are often remarkable.

Screening for infection, and treatment, should be routine for any couple experiencing problems with getting pregnant. Symptoms, when they occur, can vary in severity but generally, in women, will include an unusual discharge. This may be thicker than usual, more abundant, a different colour (ranging from yellow to greenish), and may smell bad. In addition the vaginal area might be irritated, sore and itchy and there may be a degree of cystitis. If, however, the infection is around the cervix, causing cervicitis, there may be fewer and less long-lived symptoms, especially if the infection moves upwards into the Fallopian tubes. In men the symptoms may be as limited as a discharge from the penis and a degree of cystitis.

Infection Screens for Women

Cervical Swab

Used to check for:

- Papilloma (HPV)
- Bacterial vaginosis
- Parasites
- Mixed anaerobes
- Haemophilus
- Streptococci
- Staphylococci
- Gonococcal infection (gonorrhoea)
- Mycoplasma/ureaplasma
- Candida
- Chlamydia by PCR
- Herpes Simplex Antigen, dependent on history

Blood Tests

Used to check for:

- Cytomegalovirus (CMV)
- Toxoplasma IgG and IgM
- Parvo B-19 if pregnant
- Chlamydia antibodies
- Hepatitis B surface antigen
- Syphilis (VDRL and TPHA), dependent on history

The most common causes of infection in the reproductive tract, of which some are implicated in fertility problems, are:

- Candida albicans
- chlamydia
- ureaplasma
- gonorrhoea
- bacterial vaginosis (Gardnerella)
- trichomonas vaginalis
- herpes

Let's take a closer look at each of these.

Candida

This seems to have become a bit of a buzz word – the whole country seems to have Candida! *Candida albicans* is the name of the yeast organism that exists quite normally and without problem in the gut and vagina, causing no problems – unless there is an overgrowth. This can be caused by a number of things including a generally poor diet high in refined sugars, hormone treatments (including the Pill), antibiotics (which kill off the 'good' bacteria in the gut or genito-urinary tract in both men and women that help keep Candida in check), stress and poor health. Initial symptoms are those of vaginal thrush – discharge and irritation. It is important for both partners to be treated with anti-fungal pessaries and cream, to prevent re-infection.

One problem is that a proliferation of Candida may not remain local to the vagina, causing recognizable symptoms of discharge and irritation, but may become systemic – affecting the whole body. Symptoms at this stage can include food cravings for sweet things (to 'feed' the yeast overgrowth), chronic vaginal thrush that doesn't respond to topical treatment, chronic tiredness, Irritable

Bowel Syndrome (IBS), depression, a change in bowel habits and an inability to absorb nutrients adequately. If a Candida infection becomes systemic, it is referred to as candidiasis or dysbiosis, and can be difficult to treat.

Candida species may be isolated from the genital tract of approximately 20 per cent of asymptomatic, healthy women of childbearing age. How asymptomatic colonization develops is unknown, but it can persist for years. About 75 per cent of adult women from all socio-economic strata will suffer at some point in their lives.

Some women never develop symptoms, some have intermittent episodes and others have recurrent (four or more) episodes each year or chronic infections.

Pruritis (itching) is present in virtually all cases of symptomatic vaginal and vulval Candida (VVC). This is worse at night and can be exacerbated by warmth. Other symptoms include burning vulval discomfort and superficial dyspareunia (pain during intercourse). Many patients with recurrent candidiasis experience symptoms just before the onset of their period (premenstrually); these symptoms then disappear once the period begins.

Candida in Men

Asymptomatic candidal colonization, especially in uncircumcised men is more common than the symptomatic disease. Penile candidiasis is nearly always, but not exclusively, associated with infection in the female: Candida species can cause inflammation of the glans penis and foreskin (balanoposthitis), but more often there's a transient, itchy rash, erythema (burning) that develops shortly after intercourse. These symptoms will disappear after washing.

Treatment

There are a number of things that can be done to prevent a Candida infection in the first place, or to increase the chances of controlling it once it has been diagnosed. The first step is to ensure that you reduce the amount of sugar in your diet, cutting out all refined sugars, and products made with these. Also reduce your intake of food items that contain yeast – from bread to beer – and any other fermented foods (such as yeast extract), plus cheeses made with mould – again, a yeast product. Instead, increase your intake of fresh foods, and eat 'live' yoghurt, which contains *Lactobacillus acidophilus*, every day. Taking a good quality probiotic is especially important if you have been on antibiotics. This will contain the same active ingredient as live yoghurt and will help re-colonize your gut with those 'good' bacteria that keep yeast infections like Candida at bay.

Some women seem particularly prone to repeated infections, so taking steps to reduce your risk is important. Wearing loose-fitting cotton underwear (avoiding thongs and G-strings – at our clinic the policy is 'Big knickers are best!'), and stockings rather than tights will help to keep the vaginal area cool and less moist. Wash all underwear in non-biological powders and rinse well. Add a handful of salt to the bath, or a few drops of tea tree oil (which is anti-fungal) rather than bubble bath, wash daily and make sure all soap and soap products used are rinsed off well. Also, don't over-wash: some women I see wash the area far too frequently with perfumed products.

Chlamydia

This is the most common infection treated by STI clinics. Its incidence is rising and its symptoms are often referred to as 'non-specific' because they can be rather vague. This leads to a lack of diagnosis, and the continued passing on of the bacterium (*Chlamydia trachomatis*) that causes it. CT is associated with urethral or vaginal discharge. In men, approximately 50 per cent of all chlamydial infections have no symptoms; in women this can be as high as 80 per cent. If left untreated, the infection may lead to complications such as pelvic inflammatory disease (PID) and preventable infertility in women due to the damage the infection can do to the internal reproductive organs if not treated in time.

In men, a chlamydia infection may lead to chronic prostatitis or epididymo-orchitis (inflammation of the testicles or epididymis), which is associated with reduced fertility. In some men it triggers joint pain. Having said this, Chlamydia is relatively easy to check for, either by taking a swab from the cervical area of the vagina or from the urethra in men, or by taking a urine sample. Modern nucleic acid amplification techniques (NAAT) such as the polymerase chain reaction (PCR) or strand displacement amplification have made the diagnosis of Chlamydia more sensitive. If you think it might be worth getting tested, ask your GP or make an appointment at your local clinic. Once diagnosed, Chlamydia can be treated with specific antibiotics. Always remember that any course of antibiotics must be completed, even if your symptoms seem to have cleared up completely. Taking a probiotic while on a course of antibiotics is also a good idea, as this helps avoid the possibility of coming down with vaginal thrush!

Mycoplasma and Ureaplasma

Non-gonococcal Urethritis and Salpingitis

Ureaplasma urealyticum is a cause of non-gonococcal urethritis, also known as non-specific urethritis (NGU, NSU) in men and women free of *Chlamydia trachomatis*, which is an established agent of non-gonococcal urethritis. Eighty per cent of all sexually active persons have evidence of *U. urealyticum* present and are generally symptom-free.

However, in patients with NGU there is a great deal of evidence, such as that produced by Dr Shmuel Razin, which has demonstrated that symptoms can be cured primarily on the production of non-gonococcal urethritis symptoms in ureaplasma-free and Chlamydia-free volunteers by intra-urethral inoculation of *U. urealyticum*. It has also been reported that this disease could be cured in a Chlamydia-free man only when he and his partner were treated simultaneously with tetracycline, which eliminated *U. urealyticum* from both.

Ureaplasma have also been associated with chorioamnionitis, a general term for infection of the amniotic membranes (the chorion, amnion and placenta, and sometimes also the umbilical cord) by bacteria, *Mycoplasma* and ureaplasma during pregnancy. The infection weakens the membranes, which results in premature rupture. Inflammation causes swelling around the placenta, which reduces the flow of blood and causes hypoxia in the foetus, and by-products of bacteria and/or of foetal distress initiate preterm labour, habitual spontaneous abortion and low-weight infants.

Mycoplasma hominis, a common inhabitant of the vagina in healthy women, becomes pathogenic once it invades the internal genital organs, where it may cause pelvic inflammatory abscess or salpingitis. It has been suggested that *Mycoplasma genitalium* may account for the 20 per cent of tetracycline-responsive NGU cases in which Chlamydia and ureaplasma cannot be isolated.

This infection is commonly associated with chlamydia, Candida and trichomonas infections of the reproductive systems of both men and women. Once identified, however, a course of antibiotics is generally advised, together with addressing any other, related health issues – such as poor diet, lifestyle choices, etc.

It is important to identify and treat this infection in couples trying to get pregnant – not least because studies have shown that couples experiencing fertility problems are more likely to have high concentrations of this bacterium in their genital tracts. The motility and levels of sperm in infected men can be affected, which may create problems with conception.

In addition, there is a suspected link between ureaplasma and miscarriage. Ureaplasma is routinely checked for in US clinics, because of the risk it presents if it gets into the uterus, but this is not the case in the UK.

Gonorrhoea

This is a highly infectious bacterial disease which produces complications that are especially risky for conception. As with Chlamydia, nucleic acid amplification techniques have helped with diagnosing gonorrhoea. Again, though, there can be problems with diagnosis because as many as 70 per cent of women infected have no symptoms at all, although statistically twice as many men as women are infected. Men show symptoms of discharge, high fever and abdominal pain within a week of infection. At this stage of the infection there is also a risk of meningitis, inflammation of the heart (pericarditis, myocarditis, endocarditis), hepatitis, arthritis and epididymitis (painful inflammation of the epididymes in the testes). In 20 to 40 per cent of all cases, there is a co-infection with chlamydia.

However, it is the after-affects of infection – PID (pelvic inflammatory disease) in women, causing the Fallopian tubes to block – that can have a devastating effect on fertility. Early diagnosis and treatment are essential. Of course, this can be difficult if the woman experiences no symptoms. Any man with this diagnosis will be advised to alert his most recent partners, because of the risk to their fertility.

Any course of antibiotic treatment must be given to both partners, and completed in order to avoid encouraging the emergence of resistant strains of bacteria. During this time it's advised not to participate in unprotected intercourse – use a condom until the infection is completely cleared – and re-test after 10 days' treatment to be sure you are clear before having unprotected intercourse again.

Bacterial Vaginosis (Gardnerella)

Bacterial vaginosis (BV) is probably the most common form of vaginal infection in women of reproductive age, accounting for at least a third of all vulvo-vaginal infections. Discharge is often excessive and can stain undergarments, and may have a 'fishy' odour. Some women report a connection between the onset of the discharge and a change of sexual partner – however, it is quite often the case that they have had the problem all along. The discharge is normally whitish or greyish-white; the thin discharge can be easily wiped from the vaginal walls and cervix and resembles 'flour-paste'.

Hormonal factors may play a role in this change of the environment of the vagina; we also know that seminal fluid is immunosuppressive and may have a stimulatory effect on the BV organisms. Semen also increases the vaginal pH.

There is usually a degree of vaginal irritation and vulval discomfort, and intercourse is painful as a consequence. Although not classified as an STI, bacterial vaginosis is aggravated by sexual intercourse, and while there may not be a direct impact on fertility (though there is evidence to suggest that there is an increased risk of miscarriage), it is often found in conjunction with other infections. Treatment with antibiotics may be necessary, but often it resolves itself if other factors – such as poor nutrition, the use of feminine hygiene sprays, douching, other infections, etc. – are eliminated. Men don't seem to be so susceptible to this infection, even if having unprotected intercourse with an infected woman.

Trichomonas Vaginalis

Although similar to bacterial vaginitis, trichomonas is a parasite. Most people infected are asymptomatic (show no symptoms), but when symptoms do arise they are similar to those of BV: discharge with a strong fishy odour and discomfort during intercourse. Although not implicated in fertility problems, trichomonas is sexually transmitted and can be associated with other infections, so needs proper diagnosis and treatment.

Herpes

Herpes simplex infection is far more common than you might think. Many couples have this and are very embarrassed by it, when really it is nothing to be ashamed of, as herpes is present in by far the vast proportion of the population, although in most people it lies dormant so they aren't aware of this.

Treatment Options

Most infections are treatable with antibiotics. During the course of any treatment, it's as well to support your body in its efforts by boosting your immune system. The first step is to ensure that you are eating well (see Nutrition chapter). There are also particular supplements that can give your general health a bit of a boost:

- a good-quality probiotic. Choose one that combines *Lactobacillus acidophilus* and *Bifidobacterium bifidus.*
- B vitamins – Women with vaginal infections are often found to be short on this group of vitamins.
- Garlic has effective anti-bacterial properties. Either eat lots of the natural product or find a supplement that contains the primary active ingredient in garlic: allicin.

- Zinc is vital for supporting the immune system.
- Antioxidant vitamins A, C and E are beneficial.

Having said this, rather than try to self-prescribe you should always consult a qualified nutritionist so you know the correct dose you should be taking of these and any other relevant supplements.

Menstrual Cycle

As explained in the Female Fertility chapter, your menstrual cycle can tell you a lot about your own fertility or the risk of potential problems such as lack of ovulation and hormonal problems. Later in this chapter we will also look at other possible underlying health problems that affect fertility, such as thyroid problems (see page 256) and PCOS (see page 263).

First off, you should see a doctor **before** you start trying to conceive if:

- you have problem periods: they are irregular, painful (requiring the use of painkillers), heavy, or absent
- you have a history of gynaecological infections, any abdominal surgery or a burst appendix, which could have caused pelvic inflammation and infection
- there are noticeable changes in the length of your monthly cycle
- there is spotting or bleeding between periods
- you find sexual intercourse painful in any way.

Lifestyle Factors

There are many of these that need to be considered – see the Lifestyle Factors chapter – and include everything from alcohol consumption to the use of lubricative gels, painkillers and over-the-counter medications.

Underlying Medical Disorders

One of the benefits of taking an integrated approach to fertility, for both partners, is that you are looking at the *whole picture* – this is very much my approach. For some men, being slightly overweight may not cause a problem to their fertility, for example, but in others it may be associated with poor nutrition or excessive alcohol intake and, as a consequence, poor sperm production. A woman who is constantly tired may not think this is a bar to conception, but if the cause of her tiredness is an underactive thyroid, or subclinical iron-deficiency anaemia, then these problems need addressing. Hormonal problems, which are diagnosed with blood tests, can alert your doctor to potential ovulation problems.

As outlined in earlier chapters, from the moment of first meeting a couple, and in conjunction with their very detailed questionnaires, I can sometimes pinpoint quite easily where a problem may lie and whether further investigations or help is needed.

Basic Fertility Tests

Blood tests will be the first investigation if you are having problems conceiving, and will tell your doctor if there are any problems with:

- Follicle-stimulating Hormone (FSH) levels
- Oestradiol levels
- Luteinizing Hormone (LH) levels
- Prolactin levels
- Progesterone

Additional tests can be run on a blood sample to check for:

- Full blood count
- Thyroid hormone levels
- Rubella
- Toxoplasmosis
- CMV
- Inhibin B

FSH Levels

Follicle-stimulating hormone is produced in the pituitary gland: as its name suggests, it stimulates the follicles to produce oestrogen; it also stimulates the ovary to produce an egg. The oestrogen produced then in turn affects the pituitary gland to slow down the production of FSH. This is called 'negative feedback': the effect keeps the FSH level low under normal circumstances.

The lower the FSH level, the better this will be read by your doctor on Days 1–3, in conjunction with oestradiol levels; a raised FSH level is an indication that the ovaries are beginning to struggle. As the ovaries begin to struggle, higher levels of FSH are necessary to produce the same effects.

FSH Levels

Less than 6   Excellent. Very reassuring level.

6–8   Normal. Expect a good response to stimulation.

8–10   Fair. Response is between completely normal and some-what reduced (response varies widely). Overall, a some-what reduced live birth rate.

10–12   Lower ovarian reserve. Usually shows a reduced response to stimulation and some reduction in egg and embryo quality with IVF. Reduced live birth rates.

12–17   Generally shows a more marked reduction in response to stimulation and usually a further reduction in egg and embryo quality with IVF. Low live birth rates.

Over 17   'No go.' Very poor (or no) response to stimulation. No live births. 'No go' levels must be individualized for the particular lab assay and IVF centre.

Many of the women I see, especially those in their late thirties, have a raised or high FSH level. This sends some into a complete panic, particularly as the word 'menopause' is often used in the same sentence. Raised FSH affects many women who are peri-menopausal (the name for the period of about 10 years before the menopause). When the readings get very high – in the twenties and thirties – it is an indication that you are getting closer to the menopause.

I have seen many women come to my clinic desperate following a high FSH result. Procedures vary from clinic to clinic, but some will not let you enter into an IVF programme with an FSH above 10. A lot of the women I see come to get their FSH levels down to be able to start an IVF programme – and, I'm happy to report, go on to get pregnant naturally even with an FSH of 12 to 14.

What You Can Do

There is currently no effective medical treatment for raised FSH levels, although research has shown that acupuncture can help. As a trained and practising acupuncturist, I use this treatment with many clients, including those with raised FSH levels. There are also a number of acupuncture points for reproduction and hormone regulation.

There are also a number of immediate steps that can be taken which may help reduce FSH levels. These include:

- a detox diet (see page 152)
- cutting down on daily salt intake
- drinking at least 2 litres of bottled or filtered water a day
- avoiding tea, coffee, colas and other caffeinated, sugary or carbonated drinks
- losing weight, if overweight (see page 135)
- taking regular, gentle exercise
- spending time relaxing, deep breathing, and meditating on the colour blue
- taking a daily supplement or tincture of the herb Vitex Agnus Castus, shown to be successful in some cases of raised FSH levels – should only be taken under the supervision of a medical herbalist
- taking a vitamin B complex supplement, containing at least 50 mg of B_6
- taking a zinc supplement
- taking EFAs (either evening primrose oil or DHA) daily
- eating beans, legumes, onions and garlic to help the liver break down excess oestrogens

While an abnormal FSH blood level result, showing a high baseline FSH, tends to be predictive of poor egg quality, conversely a normal result doesn't necessarily mean that egg quality is good. A significant number of women showing a normal FSH level still have eggs of poor quality, and this is particularly true of women in their forties.

A woman aged 44 having problems conceiving is not a good bet for IVF, even if her FSH level is normal, because the chances are that the quality of her eggs is declining. This is why IVF programmes have age cut-offs, and although individual programmes vary according to where you live and what's available, the cut-off point will vary. Women older than this rarely have successful outcomes from IVF using their own eggs, and donor eggs are often recommended, showing good results.

Oestradiol Levels

Oestradiol levels are read in conjunction with FSH. If they are high it may mean there is a cyst, or it may mean that the ovaries are struggling. Both the FSH and oestradiol readings (see below) are important, because sometimes the FSH reading will be low but the oestradiol reading will be high.

LH Levels

An elevated lnfeinizing hormone level may suggest PCOS (see page 263).

Prolactin Levels

Prolactin is a hormone secreted by the pituitary gland that prepares the breasts for milk production. It is available in large quantities in breast-feeding women, and it suppresses ovulation – nature's way of helping a breastfeeding mother avoid another pregnancy. However, levels are sometimes raised in non-pregnant and non-breastfeeding women, and ovulation is suppressed in a similar way.

Unsurprisingly, given its role, raised levels of prolactin cause symptoms of breast soreness and swelling, menstrual irregularities because of non-ovulation, and in some women the production of breast milk (galactorrhoea).

A rise in prolactin levels is normally caused by the hormonal feed-back towards the end of pregnancy, and during labour and birth, which stimulates a woman's milk to 'come in'. In men, who produce prolactin in small amounts, an increase in production (usually caused by a benign tumour in the pituitary gland, or by hypothyroidism) can interfere with LH activity in the Leydig cells, which slows down the production of testosterone and interferes with sperm production.

In both sexes, however, raised prolactin levels can also be caused by a drop in the secretion of a neuro-transmitter manufactured in the cortex of the brain, called dopamine. A reduction in dopamine can also cause a decrease in libido or sexual interest. Prolonged stress, which produces excessive secretion of adrenaline, causes dopamine deficiency, as can excessive exercise. In addition, raised prolactin levels can be caused by:

- drugs, including anti-depressants, blood pressure medication and anaesthetics
- opiates like cocaine
- alcohol, and particularly beer
- an underactive thyroid
- PCOS (in a woman)
- a benign growth (adenoma) of the pituitary gland

Fortunately, a raised prolactin level is easily diagnosed by a simple blood test, and can be treated medically with drugs, which work by inhibiting the secretion of prolactin by the pituitary gland.

It may also be possible to make a difference to prolactin levels by using therapies that promote deep relaxation, like massage, reflexology or meditation, all of which will reduce the effects of stress if practised regularly. Balancing this with regular – but not excessive – gentle exercise, as part of stress management, is good. A good nutritious diet, with lots of foods containing B vitamins, magnesium and zinc will help, as this improves the natural formation of dopamine. Supplementing the diet with B$_6$, zinc and magnesium may also be necessary. Avoiding alcohol and other opiates, and reviewing any anti-depressant medication, is important too.

If prolactin levels are normalized, the good news is that normal ovulation – or sperm production – will return in most cases. So, although the initial diagnosis may make for depressing news, there is a lot that can be done by the individual concerned, and much to be optimistic about.

Thyroid Problems

The thyroid is a small gland that produces hormones affecting all the metabolic processes of the body. It has a big influence on a woman's fertility as it can affect ovulation.

Thyroid problems are much more common than is often thought: about 2 per cent of the population have an underactive thyroid (also known as hypothyroidism), and 2 per cent have an overactive thyroid (hyperthyroidism). Women are affected about 10 times more frequently than men.

Thyroid problems can also be inherited, and are commonly an auto-immune condition, where antibodies are produced by the body that attack the thyroid gland. Some women develop a thyroid problem after pregnancy.

One problem in diagnosing an underactive thyroid is that it might be borderline, and show few definite symptoms.

The main cause of thyroid problems lies with the thyroid gland itself, which may just not produce enough of the necessary hormone (thyroxine). Alternatively, the feedback mechanism that stimulates the thyroid gland to secrete the right levels of hormone may be at fault, and sometimes there is a failure of the body to use the hormone correctly.

Symptoms of an underactive thyroid vary, depending on the individual, but can include some or all of the following, to a greater or lesser extent (the first seven in this list are the most common):

- tiredness, to the point of exhaustion
- sensitivity to cold
- palpitations
- period problems
- loss of libido
- weight gain or loss
- constipation
- skin problems
- joint stiffness
- PMS
- impotence (in men)
- dry hair
- alopecia (hair loss)
- brittle nails
- memory impairment
- muscle cramps
- depression.

Your menstrual cycle can offer vital clues when it comes to detecting thyroid problems. An underactive thyroid can make your periods heavier for longer and your cycle shorter. In its more severe stages, an underactive thyroid can even cause anovulation (no ovulation) and irregular periods or amenorrhoea (no periods at all).

Diagnosis is usually made by a blood test, which your GP can do. Once diagnosed, the only treatment is a daily replacement of the thyroid hormone in the form of synthetic thyroxine. Regular blood tests are also necessary to ensure that the drug treatment provided is at the right level. Too much or too little can create its own problems. So remember that even if you are diagnosed with a thyroid problem, it is treatable – women on thyroxine have reported amazing results in how much better they feel.

It is essential that any complementary treatments – and acupuncture can help, for example – are utilized in conjunction with the appropriate drug therapy. In any case of a thyroid disorder, however, ensure that your nutritional intake is good, especially if you are trying to get pregnant. Essential nutrients here include the B vitamins, Co-enzyme Q10, magnesium, calcium, selenium, zinc and iodine (see Nutrition chapter, page 55). Your diet should also include foods that contain iodine, the amino acid triosine, selenium and cystine.

There are also certain foods that inhibit thyroid function, mainly from the brassica family of vegetables – though it has to be said that these vegetables also contain important nutrients, and cooking usually deactivates the thyroid-hampering substances (known as goitrogens). You will be more susceptible to this if there is a family history of thyroid problems.

Iron-deficiency Anaemia

Anaemia describes the effect of a lack of oxygen-carrying red blood cells on the body. Every cell in the body needs an adequate supply of oxygen to function; without it the body will go into survival mode to protect the vital organs. If you are trying to get pregnant, this will affect your fertility and make conception difficult.

Oxygen binds with the pigment *haemoglobin* in red blood cells, and haemoglobin can't be produced unless there is an adequate intake of iron. It is estimated that 42 per cent of women under the age of 40, and 33 per cent of all women in the UK, are getting less iron than they need. Women are at greater risk of anaemia than men, especially during their fertile years when they are having regular periods, and some women are more prone to it than others. If you have heavy periods, this could lead to or exacerbate anaemia.

Diagnosis is made by a blood test. Healthy levels in a woman should be between 11-15 g/dl. Usually this test is done in conjunction with a full blood count so that other information about blood cells can be diagnosed. Other forms of anaemia can also be picked up in this way.

Iron in the diet is mostly easily obtained from red meat, so vegetarians can be at risk of deficiency. Numerous drugs, including antacids and antibiotics, can affect the absorption of iron, while seemingly innocuous black tea, which contains tannin, can also inhibit its absorption. Even a high dairy intake can inhibit iron absorption.

In addition, iron can only be absorbed in the presence of an adequate intake of vitamin C, which has to be taken daily as it can't be stored by the body.

Once the levels of red blood cells have fallen, it can take anything up to six weeks for them to recover. Dietary changes alone may not be sufficient, and an iron supplement may be recommended.

Many find that iron supplements can cause problems with constipation, so up your liquid and fruit juice intake (also good for vitamin C), while also ensuring that you're getting plenty of fibre in your diet.

In extreme cases of anaemia, a blood transfusion could be necessary to restore levels to normal.

Symptoms of anaemia, which will vary in severity depending on how low your levels of haemoglobin have fallen, include:

- tiredness
- breathlessness
- pale skin
- dizziness
- palpitations
- physical weakness
- susceptibility to infections.

Sometimes there might be only a few symptoms, or they might be vague, even when a person is quite anaemic.

Iron is not the only important nutrient when it comes to red blood cells. Also needed are adequate intakes of vitamin B_{12} and folic acid, plus, as mentioned, vitamin C to help with the absorption of iron.

Diabetes

Although you are unlikely to have diabetes and not know it, occasionally investigation for fertility problems can result in a diagnosis of diabetes. This is because an abnormally high level of insulin in the blood, which will affect the body's ability to tolerate glucose levels, can sometimes affect fertility hormones and result in a failure to ovulate. In addition, a woman with badly managed diabetes is six times more likely to miscarry. (See also the section on PCOS, page 263.)

Diabetes occurs when the pancreas fails to secrete enough insulin to regulate the exchange of sugar (glucose) between the blood and the body's cells. Insulin acts as a bridge between the two, making sure there is enough – but no more than that – for the cells to use for the production of energy. Without adequate glucose, body cells – for example, those in the brain – can't function properly. An excess of glucose in the body's cells, on the other hand, can also be damaging, for example to the retina of the eye.

One of the first signs of untreated diabetes is a constant thirst, combined with a need to urinate frequently and an excessive production of urine. High levels of blood sugar can also cause blurred vision and, in women, recurrent thrush infections. Infections and wounds that are slow to heal, in either men or women, are another sign, as is impotence in men.

Diabetes is a debilitating illness that can result in fatigue and a chronic lack of energy. There is a genetic component to diabetes, so if there is a history of diabetes in your family you may have a genetic predisposition to the disease. Another predisposing factor is obesity, which is thought to be the reason why there is a growing trend of what is known as Type II diabetes in children, where this type previously occurred far more often in people over the age of 55.

Treatment depends on the cause and type of diabetes. If it is mild and the body is still producing some insulin, it can be controlled by diet alone. Otherwise, insulin-replacement injections will be needed to control blood sugar levels.

If diabetes is well managed in either partner there is no reason why pregnancy shouldn't occur naturally, as long as there are no other problems. I do, however, advise anyone with diabetes who is planning a pregnancy to ensure they have expert care. The management and control of diabetes is very important during pregnancy, as women with diabetes have a greater risk of miscarriage, foetal abnormality and a tendency to give birth to large babies.

Underlying Reproductive Disorders

Among the reasons why couples fail to get pregnant are those specific disorders of the reproductive system that make conception difficult. It may be that you are aware of a health problem that might lead to difficulties in conception, or this may only become apparent when you try to conceive. For example, the symptoms of PCOS (polycystic ovary syndrome) can vary from mild to moderate to severe. In some cases the symptoms are so mild that the syndrome goes undiagnosed, while alternatively it may be something that you have struggled with for years, knowing that it might make getting pregnant difficult.

Such disorders are usually diagnosed by further investigations to check your Fallopian tubes. Dye is injected through the tubes to see if they are 'patent' (clear) or not. If they are damaged, there is an increased risk of an ectopic pregnancy. Your doctor will advise you on how to progress, and on whether you should continue to try to conceive naturally or should go straight to IVF. Women with blocked Fallopian tubes usually do well with IVF.

Further investigations would include laparoscopy, a surgical procedure to examine the health of the womb for a clear view of any fibroids, endometriosis, PCOS or structural problems.

Anovulation

During the first, follicular stage of the menstrual cycle, the main problem when it comes to fertility is no ovulation. This is generally because of inadequate secretions of FSH and LH, as well as oestrogen. It is clear that the interplay between these three hormones, which are in a delicate balance, is the key factor in ovulation.

Women who have an irregular cycle don't always ovulate. A very long or short follicular (pre-ovulatory) phase can influence the overall length of the cycle, causing it to fluctuate in length from cycle to cycle. This can indicate that there are some hormonal balances that need adjusting.

Adjusting hormonal balance for fertility can be done in a variety of ways. I use acupuncture, but diet also has a role to play, as do exercise, hypnosis and stress-reduction techniques (see page 183).

If you are not ovulating, you also need to work in conjunction with Western medicine, particularly if absent or very light periods have been common throughout your menstrual history, or if your weight may be a factor.

Period Problems

Amenorrhoea

Amenorrhoea is an absence of periods. This is common in women who have just come off the Pill. It can also be linked to weight loss and over-exercising.

Dysmenorrhoea

This is the term used to describe very heavy and painful periods. This can lead to further problems such as anaemia or the overuse of painkillers. Nutrition (including supplements), diet, acupuncture and Western medical techniques can all help.

PCOS

With PCOS, the ovaries produce imbalanced levels of hormonal secretions, so instead of stimulating one follicle to produce one mature egg during the course of a woman's cycle, numerous follicles are inappropriately stimulated but can't mature, so form tiny cysts. These numerous cysts on the surface of the ovary can be seen clearly on an ultrasound scan. Their presence, in turn, further disrupts any hormonal secretions. Without the right hormonal environment, the possibility of ovulating a mature egg capable of being fertilized is reduced, as are the chances of implantation.

The reasons for PCOS aren't clear cut. While some think the problem originates in the hypothalamus in the brain, mastermind of reproductive hormones, other theories suggest it is a problem in the ovaries. As sometimes it is only one ovary that is affected, this may well be the case. Recent evidence points to an underlying insulin sensitivity playing a major role in the condition. High levels of insulin stimulate the ovaries, resulting in excessive androgen levels and anovulation.

What is clear is that the resulting hormone levels – of oestrogens, androgens, luteinizing hormone, etc. – cause internal havoc, not just to the reproductive organs but to other body systems. The increased production of insulin leads to blood sugar fluctuations, while an excess of androgens leads to the distressing symptom (in a woman) of facial hair. Acne is often a problem, too. You need to work in conjunction with your doctor.

Once in this vicious circle of hormonal havoc, it's difficult to feel you can exert any control over it. In fact, there is a lot that can be done to rebalance your hormones and improve your chances of conceiving.

First of all, do what you can to rebalance your blood sugar levels (see page 108) by choosing slow-release carbohydrates that have a low glycaemic index. This will help reduce the fluctuating levels of insulin and blood sugar. Make sure you eat some form of protein with any carbohydrate, as this will help to balance blood sugar levels. By looking closely at dietary factors such as this, it may also be possible to lose weight if you are overweight – often a problem with women with PCOS. Even if you are only 10 per cent over your recommended weight, this can have an impact on your fertility, especially if other health factors are involved, too. And remember: adjusting your eating habits gradually over a period of time is a far more effective way to sustain weight loss than a crash diet, which is nutritionally unsound in most cases.

In terms of nutrition, ensuring that your diet contains the recommended amount of fruits and vegetables, cutting down on animal fats while increasing your intake of essential fatty acids, and taking a good vitamin and mineral supplement should also help.

The way that we treat PCOS at the clinic is to work very much with weight loss. Studies have shown losing 10 per cent of weight can bring back normal ovulation in women with PCOS. We encourage a gradual weight loss of 2 lb a week, through diet and exercise. It is worth mentioning, however, that it is harder for women with PCOS to lose weight because the syndrome makes their bodies store fat more efficiently and burn calories more slowly. Also, some women with PCOS make the mistake of cutting out carbs completely. If you cut out carbs you will have low serotonin levels and are likely to become depressed.

The key issues we concentrate on when treating women with PCOS are:

1. blood sugar and insulin resistance
2. weight and weight loss programme
3. working with clients who are already taking drugs such as clomid and metformin and supporting any drug/nutrient interactions
4. stress and hormonal balance
5. emotional factors
6. poor body image, low self-esteem and low libido
7. sex and relationship difficulties.

In my practice, I also recommend and provide acupuncture for women with PCOS. More research has been carried out on the effect of acupuncture on PCOS than on any other gynaecological problem, and it seems that its effectiveness has to do with acupuncture's ability to stimulate B-endorphins in the body, which affect levels of GnRH (gonadotrophin-releasing hormone) and, as result, help stabilize levels of FSH (follicle-stimulating hormone) and LH (luteinizing hormone). Acupuncture has long been successful at rebalancing hormones, which in turn regulates the fertility cycle.

Regular exercise, too, will increase your metabolic rate (helping you to burn calories more efficiently), lift your spirits and energize you. This doesn't need to be a heavy-duty session at the gym every day: a brisk 20-minute walk every day will make a huge difference over time.

Exercise also helps to reduce stress levels, which is also important for women with PCOS because stress stimulates the production of more hormones, including testosterone, from the adrenals, which will further aggravate the problem. Select those stress-management techniques – yoga, meditation, swimming or just listening to music by candlelight in a scented bath every night – that work for you, and make sure you factor some relaxation into every day.

Remember that having PCOS does not mean you will never get pregnant: as many as 70 per cent of women with PCOS will get pregnant without drugs, and a further 20 per cent will conceive with assisted fertility or other treatment.

Herbal Treatment for PCOS

Herbs such as agnus castus, saw palmetto and black cohosh can be useful in treating PCOS, but must be taken under the advice of a qualified medical herbalist. At our clinic we only use them after looking at blood profiles to check various hormone levels and see if clients are eligible to take herbs. Just because a product is natural does not mean that it doesn't have potent side-effects that may compound any fertility or other health problem.

Endometriosis

This merits a book all to itself! Endometriosis is a complex disorder of the female reproductive tract, where tiny pieces of the endometrium (lining of the womb) 'migrate' to other areas in the abdomen. The problem then is that they are subject to the same hormonal fluctuations as the lining of the womb: they respond to the hormonal stimulus to thicken and produce a good blood supply, and they bleed during a period. As this is often happening in a confined space, without the outlet of the cervix and the vagina, these pieces of endometrial tissue can swell and engorge, causing pain and increasing risk of adhesions (scar tissue) and blockages.

If endometriosis is advanced and far-reaching – which can be the case, particularly as a woman grows older – it can reduce her chances of conception. While the cause of endometriosis is poorly understood, there seems to be a family link, so if your mother or sister suffers from it, your risk may be increased. This link most likely has something to do with the underlying hormonal causes of endometriosis. It is also thought that immune factors come into play.

An estimated 4 to 17 per cent of women are thought to have a degree of endometriosis, which can vary from mild to moderate to severe. Pain, especially during a period (which may be heavy and last for up to a week), is often a significant indicator, although without laparoscopic investigations (where a fibre-optic tube is passed into the abdominal cavity to check the internal reproductive organs) it can be difficult to make a definitive diagnosis.

The severity of symptoms does not reflect the severity of the condition, as there may be no symptoms at all or a combination of several types, including:
- severe pain and cramping
- pain during intercourse
- spotting between periods
- heavy periods
- PMS.

As to the causes, there are many different theories (see Nutrition chapter, page 115).

Fibroids

Fibroids are an overgrowth of the myometrium, the middle, muscular layer of the womb. Fibroids can grow quite large, thus preventing implantation of a fertilized egg. They are benign tumours, and only very rarely – in 0.5 per cent of cases – do they become malignant. Although growing from the muscular layer of the womb, rather than the endometrium, they too can respond to hormonal changes during a woman's cycle. In some women their presence causes heavy bleeding and pain (menorrhagia) during a period. Because of this, they can cause anaemia in some women, leaving them very tired and prone to infections.

It is estimated that between 20 and 50 per cent of women aged between 35 and 50 have fibroids, making them the most common structural abnormality of the womb. If large enough they can be felt by the doctor (abdominal palpation), and may even cause pressure on the bladder, creating symptoms such as an urgent and/or frequent need to urinate.

Whether or not fertility is affected by fibroids depends largely on their size, and where they grow. Occasionally, fibroids can grow outside the womb. If fibroids are small they won't necessarily interfere with conception or fertilization – many women give birth successfully in spite of the presence of small fibroids.

As fibroids are oestrogen sensitive, many women find adopting a low-fat, high-fibre, mostly vegetarian diet can help. If there is excessive bleeding, and the possibility of anaemia, taking an iron supplement (in conjunction with vitamin C to help absorption, see page 129) is advisable. Other supplements that can be helpful are vitamin B, vitamin E, calcium, magnesium and potassium, and the amino acid methionine.

You may be more at risk of fibroids if there is a family history of them – if your mother or sister suffered. If surgery is advocated for their removal, there are a number of different procedures. A myomectomy simply removes the fibroids surgically, either via the vagina or through the abdomen, depending on their size. For those concerned about the effects on their fertility, you will need to consider, with your GP/health-care provider, the treatments available to you.

Immune System Problems

In my practice over the last four or five years, the number of women being diagnosed with some category or other of immune problems has steadily increased. Immune problems may contribute to recurrent pregnancy loss, family history of miscarriage, three or more IVF failures, endometriosis, auto-immune disorders, lupus, rheumatoid arthritis, Crohn's Disease, chronic fatigue syndrome (also known as M.E.), skin rashes and hives, as well as thyroid problems (overactive or underactive). The medical establishment is divided over this whole area of medicine, with few agreeing on treatment. This leaves clients confused, often feeling that they have to be virtually doctors themselves to understand the treatments and drugs available and to make decisions about embarking on expensive drugs with different side-effects. However, I have seen their use make a big difference to many clients: women who have had miscarriages or failed IVF have gone on to conceive successfully after treatment. Work is continuing in the field of reproductive immunology, and particularly on the links between the immune system and recurrent miscarriages, fertility problems and failures of IVF treatment.

Immune Problems Relating to Fertility

- Thyroid antibodies (see page 256)
- Antiphospholipids (APLAs, see page 271)
- Anti-nuclear antibodies (ANAs, see page 271)
- Natural Killer cells (see page 272)

The reason the immune system is important to fertility has to do with the delicate interplay between different immune cells and the way they work for and against us. A woman's ability to host a pregnancy depends upon complex and sophisticated immunological adjustments.

In addition, the drugs used to treat immune problems can be powerful and nothing is known as yet about their possible long-term effects. All of this has contributed to the controversy in the medical profession surrounding reproductive immunology.

To understand the complexities of the immune system, you can compare it to an army. Each part of the immune army has its own function, and each part helps the others in what they are trying to do. Its main aim is to kill off invaders, and different cells have different functions – some work on 'surveillance' while others are programmed to kill. In order for the troops to move about to where they are needed, you need to have a healthy lymphatic system. The lymphatic system is composed of glands and lymph vessels which act as a main highway throughout the body along which the white blood cells can travel to the sites which are being threatened. The long bones of our bodies produce over 2,000 immune cells per second, so it is important to keep these bones healthy and well nourished. The gut is another important station for these troops: a large percentage of the immunoglobulins are made in the gut. This is why part of my immune programme uses manual lymphatic drainage (MLD, see page 145) to help improve circulation of the lymph and support the digestive system.

There are 30 different types of white blood cells (which are called leukocytes). One type, called macrophages (the word means 'big eaters'), gobbles up all of the rubbish from our cells. These macrophages are present in large numbers in the uterus during menstruation, to clean up the uterus. In order to work well, the macrophages need an adequate supply of calcium, B vitamins and selenium.

Immune problems can take several forms: sperm may be neutralized by the woman's antibodies, the fertilized egg may not implant, or the placenta may be damaged so that the pregnancy is lost in an early miscarriage. The complex and subtle nature of immune problems, and their impact on the very early stages of conception and pregnancy, have made diagnoses difficult in the past, accounting for the number of cases of 'unexplained' infertility. Happily, with continued research, more and more couples are able to find a reason for their apparent inability to conceive, and receive appropriate treatment.

APLAs

Antiphospholipid antibodies cause problems because they increase the 'stickiness' of phospholipids – a normal part of every body cell – making them stick together. When this occurs in the placenta, damage is caused to the placental blood vessels, leading to clotting and a reduction of blood flow, so reducing the supply of oxygen and nutrients for the growing baby. APLAs can also prevent implantation, but if this occurs the damage does not reveal itself until later on, often resulting in early miscarriage.

Treatment for this is to give anti-coagulent (anti-clotting) drugs such as heparin or low-dose aspirin. Aspirin can cross the placenta, so a low dose is needed. Because aspirin can also deplete folic acid and cause loss of vitamin C, supplementation with these nutrients is also recommended. It is also important to remember that, in high doses, some supplements may thin the blood – for example, garlic, fish oils and vitamin E.

ANAs

Anti-nuclear antibodies (ANAs) will attack the nucleus of the fertilized egg, which contains all the genetic material that regulates the function of the cell. This may occur in women who already have the auto-immune disease Systemic Lupus Erythematosus (SLE). Rheumatoid arthritis – another auto-immune disease – may also be associated with the production of ANAs. If ANAs are diagnosed, the usual treatment is with corticosteroids such as dexamethaxone or prednisolone, to suppress the inflammatory response. This can help prevent the placenta becoming inflamed and weakened.

If you are diagnosed with ANAs, and prescribed corticosteroids for this problem, it's worth considering the various side-affects, which can be eased by eating the right foods. For example, ANAs reduce the activation of vitamin D, so supplementing with calcium and magnesium is recommended. Prednisolone can affect your blood sugar levels, so try and include lots of low glycaemic foods (see page 112) in your diet; many doctors also recommended regular urine testing. You should also take a good prenatal supplement complete with adequate levels of vitamin B$_6$, zinc, vitamin C and folic acid.

NK Cells

A sub-group of white blood cells are aggressive fighters: these are coded according to the type of protein-molecule receptors (clusters of differentiation, sometimes referred to as 'cd') they possess. This coding defines their function. The aggressive fighters cd16 and cd56 are known as Natural Killer cells. While their name can be frightening at first, it is these NK cells that can fight off critical illness such as cancers. We all produce NK cells (they make up 50 per cent of all white blood cells) designed to target rapidly growing and dividing cells that can cause damage.

NK cells are naturally present in the womb lining during the second half of your menstrual cycle, and promote embryo implantation by releasing substances called cytokines.

However, some NK cells are toxic to the placenta. In some women the levels of these toxic NK cells are elevated, requiring drugs (usually steroids) to dampen down their response and allow an embryo to implant successfully.

Drugs used to treat immune problems

As mentioned earlier, steroids and heparin can be used as treatments for different immune problems. Intravenous immunoglobulin (IVIg), a sterile protein derivative of blood, and an active component of immunity, is another treatment. It is given as an intravenous infusion, straight into a vein, and works in a number of ways to counteract the effects of antibodies that might otherwise inhibit the embryo's implantation:

- it suppresses the activity of NK cells
- it reduces the activity of T cells, produced normally in response to 'foreign bodies' in the body, which can damage the early implantation of the embryo
- it suppresses the production of damaging auto-antibodies, for example APLAs
- it also contains other antibodies that counteract the damaging effects of auto-antibodies.

However, it has to be mentioned that there is huge controversy around the use of IVIg, with the medical establishment divided over its efficacy.

An Immune-boosting Programme

I believe that stress, diet, lifestyle and environment all play a part in problems with the immune system, and the work I do integrates Western medicine with complementary therapies to address each of these factors:

- Detox – takes the pressure off the body's daily fight against toxins and stimulants such as caffeine, MSG, aspartame, etc., all of which can set off allergic reactions and/or cause an over-reaction on the part of the immune system. A detox can

---

also help with achieving an acid-alkaline balance – see page 113 – and gives your body a chance to build up depleted energy reserves.

- Supplements – Many women are deficient in vital vitamins and minerals, particularly those such as vitamins C and E and folic acid, which support the immune system.
- Lifestyle – alcohol, smoking, long hours, refined foods, sugar, etc. all have serious negative effects on the immune system.
- Stress – zaps your immune army. Continued or long-term stress makes your adrenal glands produce more and more cortisol, which suppresses your immune system and reduces the levels of T-helper cells. These cells affect how your body accepts a pregnancy. Stress-management techniques like hypnotherapy and meditation can really help.

Problems Affecting Men's Fertility

Over the last 50 years there has been a worldwide reduction in average sperm counts, from 113 million per ml, to 70 million per ml. Not only that, but the percentage of sperm being produced with abnormalities has gone up 12-fold, and sperm motility has deteriorated. Recent research suggests there is a general decline in sperm production, by up to 50 per cent in some men. Given this information, it's well worth every man reviewing how his health might affect sperm production, so that he can make lifestyle choices that will improve his and his partner's chances of conceiving.

In a lot of cases there is so much that can be done to improve sperm health. Men produce sperm 24 hours a day, 7 days a week. Lifestyle improvements, nutrition and antioxidants can really help improve the sperm.

It is worth considering expert advice if you have:

- had the mumps, followed by testicular inflammation
- any history of sexually transmitted infection like NSU or gonorrhoea
- undescended testicles
- problems with intercourse such as premature ejaculation or sustaining an erection
- repeated exposure to environmental hazards, chemicals or radiation without adequate protection.

Screening and Analysis

While the work being done in the field of male fertility is very exciting and we are getting very good results, two things are worth bearing in mind:

1. Semen analysis should always be done in a specialist clinic.
2. Sexual health screens: Many couples have infections they do not know about, which can impact on fertility. Some of the more routine checks can be done at local hospitals that have a genito-urinary clinic, though very often the tests are basic and do not include screening for infections that can affect fertility.

Infection Screens for Men

Urine Analysis

First urination of the day, mid-stream urine and/or prostatic massage urine are checked for:

Number of white cells and red cells per high per field (HPF)

Chlamydia by PCR

Prostatic Fluid/Swab and Semen Culture

Checked for:

- Fructose (semen only)
- Papilloma virus (HPV)
- Parasites
- Mixed anaerobes
- Haemophilus
- Streptococci
- Staphylococci
- Gonococcal infection (gonorrhoea)
- Mycoplasma ureaplasma

Other tests available will include those for:

- Candida
- Cytomegalovirus
- Hepatitis B surface antigen
- Syphilis (VDRL TPHA), dependent on history
- Herpes simplex antigen (again, will depend on history)

Case History: Jeremy and Alison

Aged 33, Jeremy and Alison had been trying to have a baby for over six years. They'd had four failed ICSI attempts (see page 336), and all the emphasis had been on Alison. Jeremy's sperm were low in everything. When they came along to our clinic, we focused on Jeremy. The first thing we did was to give him a full sexual fertility health screen, which included prostatic massage. He was found to have pus in his prostate – which may sound abnormal but is found in many of the men we see. After antibiotics, lifestyle changes and good antioxidants for four months, Jeremy and Alison conceived naturally.

The starting point for male fertility screening is the sperm test, or semen analysis. It is often offered before any other testing because it is, for the man, non-invasive and very straightforward to carry out.

Of course any sort of test can provoke a bit of anxiety, and there may be some ambivalence among men about having it done. But there is one very good reason for an early semen analysis, regardless of whether there is any degree of infertility in the woman: if an initial analysis indicates a low quantity and quality of sperm, taking steps to improve it straight away can only be beneficial.

For a comprehensive review of male reproductive health, you should also expect the sperm test to be taken in the context of a general health check. The doctor who requests the test should take a full medical history from you, including any recent illnesses and any medication that is being taken regularly, plus a sexual history, and carry out a physical check-up. Once the sample has been provided, results are available pretty quickly, so making a follow-up appointment then and there to discuss the results is a good idea.

If the initial semen analysis highlights a severe problem, a hormone

Patient Name		Difficulty producing sample?	
Name of Partner		Was all the sample collected?	
Date of Sample		Is patient on medication?	

		Reference WHO 1999
Duration of abstinence (days)		2–7 days
Interval between ejaculation and start of analysis (min)		≤ 2 hrs
Macroscopic Examination		
Volume (ml)		≥ 2 mls
Appearance		Normal
Liquefaction		Complete
Viscosity		Normal
pH		7.2–8.0
Debris		
Agglutination		
Motility (% spermatozoa)		≥ 50% (a + b); ≥ 25% (a)
(a) rapid progression		
(b) slow progression		
(c) non-progressive		
(d) immotile		
Vitality (% live)		> 50%
Antisperm Antibodies (% with adherent particles)		< 50% may not affect fertility
MAR test for IgA		
MAR test for IgG		
Concentration (x 10^6/ml)		
Count/ml		≥ 20 x 10^6/ml
Total count in ejaculate		≥ 40 x 10^6
Other Cells (x 10^6/ml)		
round cells		<5 x 10^6/ml
white blood cells		<1 x 10^6/ml
Morphology (%)		Multicentre studies in progress
normal		≥ 15%
abnormal		
head defects		

assessment may be the next step, done from a blood sample. Following this, further tests might include ultrasound scanning, biopsy, genetic tests and a more detailed physical examination, depending on what has been revealed by previous tests.

Providing a Sample

Providing a sample of semen for analysis is done by masturbating to ejaculation and collecting this in a sterile container, after which the semen is examined under a microscope. This can be done at home, if you can get the sample to the lab within an hour. Alternatively, clinics provide a room where this can be done in complete privacy. However, a lot of men feel embarrassed and uncomfortable about this, especially as in some cases men find it impossible in the clinical surroundings of a hospital to come up with the goods. I can certainly understand this, and feel sorry for men having to 'perform' in a small room while people mill about just the other side of the door! The other option, which can also be helpful for men for whom masturbation is against their religious beliefs, is to use a non-spermicidal, non-latex condom during sex, and then get the sample directly to the lab.

It's also worth remembering that semen is affected by extreme cold, so care needs to be taken, especially in winter, to keep the semen at body temperature on this journey to the lab.

It's customary to ask a man to avoid ejaculating for two to five days prior to producing a sample. In some cases, a urine sample, to be taken shortly after ejaculation, may also be requested. This is to check for a problem called 'retrograde ejaculation', which can be a factor in conception problems. Retrograde ejaculation happens when the muscular contractions of orgasm push the semen backwards into the bladder, rather than forwards to the erect penis. This muscular inefficiency is often caused by previous damage to the nerves in the area, which then convey the wrong message to the muscles. Diabetes can cause this, as can paraplegia and surgery to the prostate. However, it is possible to recover sperm from the bladder and use them for assisted conception to achieve a pregnancy.

One thing that is essential, when it comes to semen analysis, is that it is carried out properly. The analysis must be done in a specialist andrology lab. Routine pathology or microbiology labs may not have the expertise for proper assessment of the sample, and may lead to inadequate, false or misleading results. Make sure that your doctor – and at this point it is probably your GP – refers you to a specialist laboratory, well equipped to examine and interpret your sample.

Another essential point to bear in mind is that, because sperm quality is easily affected by all sorts of things, from your health to diet and stress, then even if the first result is poor, take steps to improve it and get it checked out again in three months' time. Even if it is pronounced normal, or borderline, you may be recalled for further testing over the next few months, but bear in mind the 100-day cycle for sperm improvement, and don't be in too much of a hurry to re-test.

The Results

Like most things medical, these will need some explaining, and your doctor should go through your results with you and your partner (even if they are better than normal!). Generally though, what is being looked for is that:

- at least 15 per cent of the sperm are normally shaped
- at least 50 per cent should be actively moving
- the volume of semen should be around 2ml
- there should be at least 20 million sperm per ml.

This is just a very simple summary. A full test will provide a much more comprehensive picture.

The next few pages give details of some of these factors.

A man's normal fertility can fluctuate, and is always a matter of degree. If there is a degree of sub-fertility, where the sperm count is borderline, for example, the reassuring news is that it can usually be improved. It's also important to remember that fertility is not the same as virility – an infertile man can continue to be extremely virile, for example after a vasectomy.

Identifying whether there is a problem, and to what degree, enables couples to define what their parameters of fertility are, and work with that information – whether that means major lifestyle changes, or exploring assisted conception.

IUI (intra-uterine insemination) may be helpful for men whose semen parameters fall slightly outside the reference range (between 10 and 20 million/ml, for example), and where a sperm preparation can yield more than 1 million actively progressing sperm. If the sperm show poor motility, a low count or high abnormal forms, or any combination of these, or if three or four consecutive IUI treatments have not worked, then IVF may be more appropriate.

ICSI would be advised if your sperm count is less than 5 million/ml, where motility is extremely poor or where there are fewer than 5 per cent normal forms.

Appearance

The normal appearance of sperm is greyish and slightly iridescent, and slightly sticky in nature. If it has a yellowish tinge, this can indicate a high intake of vitamin supplements, while high levels of flavoproteins result from a long abstinence from ejaculation, which is easily remedied.

More rarely, this high level of flavoproteins may indicate jaundice, but there would probably be other symptoms if this were the case.

Infection can cause a sample to have a reddish appearance, because of red blood cells, which would need investigation and treatment.

Volume

The normal amount of ejaculate in a sample is around 2 ml, or half a teaspoon. Higher than this results in a dilution in the concentration of sperm, which can affect conception. An amount of less than 1 ml can suggest a past or current infection, for example a sexually transmitted infection (STI) that has blocked the ducts that produce seminal fluid. Retrograde ejaculation (see above) can also result in low volume.

If there is low volume, and no sperm, this would suggest a physical problem like the complete absence of the vas deferens, a rare congenital abnormality with which some boys are born, often referred to as CBAVD (congenital bi-lateral absence of vas deferens). Alarming though this abnormality sounds, sperm may still be produced perfectly adequately; they're just not being ejaculated. Assisted conception remains a possibility through the surgical removal of sperm cells and insertion into a woman's egg.

Viscosity and Liquefaction

Semen has a unique ability to change its composition from being quite viscous at the point of ejaculation to becoming liquefied after about 10 minutes. This is essential for providing sperm with an alkaline and watery medium through which they can swim up through the cervix en route to an egg. If the liquefaction is poor, and is inhibiting conception, then a sperm sample can be washed and mixed with a suitable solution that allows for normal activity of the sperm before being inserted into the uterus to continue their journey.

Acidity (pH)

The pH of semen is normally quite alkaline, thanks to the secretions of the prostate gland, and this helps protect sperm from the acidity of the vagina. The pH of semen is expected to be between 7.2 and 8. A semen sample that is acidic, and without sperm, suggests an absence of the vas deferens.

Agglutination

When cells of any sort stick together, it's called agglutination, and this can happen with sperm, stopping their movement. When agglutination is seen in semen analysis, it usually indicates the presence of antibodies – produced by the man, whose immune system has incorrectly identified the sperm as 'foreign' and seeks to destroy them. Proteins from the antibodies can coat the sperm and bind them to the cervical mucus in a woman's vaginal tract. This prevents sperm travelling towards the egg.

Antibodies

When antibodies affect fertility, it is known as *immunological infertility.* The production of antibodies that affect sperm can follow surgery for hernia repair or vasectomy reversal, for example, where during surgery fragments of sperm protein may have entered the bloodstream, alerting the immune system to this 'foreign body'. If antibodies are produced in enough quantity, affecting over 50 per cent of the sperm, fertility can be affected.

While antibodies can cause agglutination, this is not the only problem that can arise. The heads of sperm can become coated with antibodies, and this can prevent sperm recognizing an egg. However, the tests for antibodies are expensive, and are not done routinely until other factors have been ruled out.

MAR (Mixed Agglutination Reaction)

This is the test used to check for antibodies, but is seldom part of a standard NHS semen analysis so you may have to ask for it, or arrange to have it done privately. If the test shows a level of binding that falls below 50 per cent, then fertility shouldn't be affected – as long as all other aspects of the semen analysis are fine.

If the binding level is over 50 per cent there are a number of treatment options to consider, including steroid treatment and assisted conception.

Round Cell Concentration

If there are round cells present in the semen, these can be either immature sperm cells or white blood cells. An excess of white blood cells can indicate an infection, which will need to be cultured for identification and treated with a course of the appropriate antibiotics. If the infection is severe, or long-standing, then there may be permanent damage to the delicate seminiferous tubules, affecting the quantity and quality of sperm.

Sperm Concentration

This aspect of semen analysis provides what most people understand by the term 'sperm count': the number of sperm present in a sample of semen. The average count nowadays is around 60-80 million per ml, although 20 million per ml is considered adequate. There is a great deal of research-based evidence that shows that sperm count is hugely affected by lifestyle factors: diet, alcohol, stress levels, exercise, infection, tobacco and recreational drugs, all of which can play havoc with sperm production. Reviewing these, and making changes, may be all that's necessary to improve production.

The complete absence of sperm in a semen sample is referred to, medically, as azoospermia, while a count of fewer than 20 million per ml is called oligozoospermia. A level of fewer than 5 million per ml can suggest a chromosomal abnormality, which may cause a woman to miscarry repeatedly.

If the count is very low, or nil, then blood tests for hormonal assessment or a testicular biopsy will probably be recommended.

Motility

To be motile is to be capable of motion. The body of a sperm contains an energy source which makes sperm capable of independent motion. Motility is a measure of the sperm's ability to move, which is a very important aspect of healthy sperm. An essential part of semen analysis is to check the ability of sperm to move quickly and in a straight line.

The motility of sperm can be affected by lifestyle factors and the frequency of ejaculation. After a long period of abstinence there will be a higher proportion of dead and immotile sperm in a sample of semen. The motility of sperm is graded in four ways, and this is referred to as progression:

a) Rapid progression is where healthy sperm move at a good speed and in straight lines.
b) Slow progression shows movement, but it is erratic and poor.
c) Non-progressive motility describes sperm that are showing slight, twitchy movements but not moving forwards.
d) Immotile refers to sperm that don't move at all.

In any sample of semen you would expect to find a mix of sperm motility. A sample of normal, fertile sperm would include at least 50 per cent of categories a) and b) described above, or 25 per cent of category a). Where the analysis falls mainly into categories c) and d), you would expect a man to have a fertility problem that could prevent conception. The technical term for poor sperm motility is asthenozoospermia.

It's worth mentioning here that heavy alcohol use can seriously affect sperm motility. While many think that the occasional alcoholic bender won't have much affect, this is a mistaken belief, and excessive alcohol intake can in fact affect the quality of a man's sperm for up to three months.

Morphology

This describes the quality of the sperm, identified by the degree of abnormalities present. These abnormalities are divided into those affecting different parts of the sperm: the head, neck, mid-piece, and tail. Abnormalities can include irregularly shaped, large or small heads (and remember, the heads carry the genetic material) – even two-headed sperm sometimes occur. Tails can be non-existent, or coiled and ineffective.

The World Health Organization (WHO) defines normal fertility as having a minimum of 15 per cent normal sperm. If a man's level of normal sperm in a sample of semen falls below this, there is likely to be a degree of sub-fertility, and where it falls below 5 per cent, a severe problem.

Where there is a high percentage of abnormal sperm, the medical term is teratozoospermia. This can be caused by lifestyle factors and, occasionally, genetic defects. Age can also play a part: after the age of 40 the number of abnormal sperm increases, although if the percentage of normal sperm remains at or over 15 per cent of the sample, then all other things being equal there shouldn't be a problem.

DNA Fragmentation

I think that this test is going to become commonplace in clinics in the next few years. We are starting to get a new breed of men through the clinic who want answers, especially if they have had failed ICSI attempts.

This test should be used if you have never fathered a child and have had failed ICSI attempts. Although it is still considered quite controversial in the UK, it is commonplace in many American clinics.

Advances in semen analysis mean that not only can the quantity and quality of sperm be assessed, but also its genetic material (DNA). Genetic abnormalities in an embryo are one of the major causes of early miscarriage. While this was previously thought to be a fault with the woman's egg, or a random mutation, it's now becoming increasingly evident that chromosomal abnormalities in sperm – which can now be screened for – can be a major contributing factor. The egg can cope with low levels of DNA damage to the sperm, but if the damage is too great the egg cannot compensate.

While genetic abnormalities can be inherited, they can also be caused by environmental factors. The major culprits behind DNA damage are free radicals from our diet and lifestyle (see page 131).

Sperm are particularly vulnerable to this because they are in constant production – but again, the good news is that this means that making the relevant changes can have a big and positive impact.

Standard sperm testing doesn't yet include checking for DNA fragmentation as routine. DNA is the genetic material within the chromosomes of sperm cells. If there are errors in this material or damage to it, for example in the structural arrangement of the cells, this can make conception difficult.

In a normally fertile man, between 2 and 13 per cent of sperm are genetically abnormal. Age has an impact on the amount of genetically abnormal material carried by sperm, while research has shown that caffeine, alcohol, cigarette smoking and exposure to environmental pollutants significantly increase the percentage of abnormality.

Currently, this test is done frequently in the US but is available only from certain clinics in the UK.

Getting a Poor Result

This is where it goes wrong for so many couples. Words like 'abnormal heads', 'only solution ICSI' can make anyone feel panicky and at a loss as to how to proceed. Make sure you don't just settle for an analysis; insist that any underlying factors are investigated fully.

Very often couples come to me confused about their results. We investigate further and get a complete picture, and see how we can improve upon the results. If the problem is genetic, there really is no chance and other avenues such as a sperm donor may be the answer.

Men can of course feel devastated, and the support they receive from their partner at this time can greatly affect how he will cope with the news. Men can feel that they have to be the strong, supportive ones, and will not talk openly even to friends. Many men crave physical and emotional support and reassurance; even though very often they are defensive and may shrug you off at first. They need to know that you still love them no matter what. When a woman is preoccupied in her pursuit to have a baby, she may not always provide her partner with the support he needs.

> *Before my results, I never thought that there was nothing I couldn't achieve or was capable of. The impact has been a loss of confidence in everything I do.*
>
> *I felt my heart sink sitting in the GP's surgery, getting the results. I was trying to keep everything together and show no emotion for my partner's sake. I could only hear certain words like 'slim chance ... ICSI'. I had always assumed that it was my partner's problem, as she had had endometriosis. I wanted to cry but couldn't. I kept thinking maybe there was a mistake. I left feeling bad, and freakish, inadequate, confused. I couldn't wait to get out of the surgery. I offered my wife a divorce.*

Don't let your sex life suffer. Couples often feel they are not going to bother to have sex because it won't 'work'. I know it can sometimes seem hopeless, but even facing results such as this, couples do go on to conceive.

A Word about Testicular Cancer

Sometimes I see couples where the male partner has had cancer in the past. Chemotherapy does halt sperm production, but in 50 per cent of cases sperm levels increase for 24 to 36 months after treatment has ended, returning to normal levels.

miscarriage

Although miscarriage isn't the same as an inability to conceive, its outcome is effectively the same – no baby – so its emotional effect on a woman and her partner can be devastating.

All women are different: some will be able, relatively soon, to come to terms with having had a miscarriage; others will take longer to heal emotionally. Once you have experienced a miscarriage, subsequent pregnancies may cause even more anxiety than normal. You lose your innocence, in some ways, and can be all too aware of the fragility of an early pregnancy. This can add to your already-raised stress levels just when rest and relaxation are what you need most.

In many ways, miscarriage is a relatively common occurrence. Most of us know a woman who has miscarried, while many women miscarry before even realizing they are pregnant. In recent years we have gained a greater understanding of the causes of miscarriage; nevertheless the experience for the majority of women remains that they have to have had three miscarriages before their doctor will refer them for further tests.

The bald statistics make depressing reading if you are a woman who has suffered one or more miscarriages. However, I genuinely believe that with the advances made through the work of experts like Professor Lesley Regan and others, identifying the causes of miscarriage is becoming better and there is an improved understanding of the role men's health may play. So again, it is important to consider both members of a couple, rather than just the woman, in determining the reasons behind a miscarriage.

In my clinic, I see that by providing couples with information, appropriate testing and details of the dietary and lifestyle changes necessary for both partners, it is absolutely possible to help increase the chances of a healthy pregnancy and baby. For couples who have experienced recurrent miscarriage, I am also of the belief that the combination of improving nutritional status before pregnancy and looking at lifestyle factors in early pregnancy can make a big difference. I always recommend a good multi-vitamin and -mineral supplement, as this one simple measure has been shown to reduce the risk of miscarriage.

How Common Is It?

Roughly half of all eggs that are fertilized never continue to implantation or, if they do, to a viable pregnancy. It's in these cases that women may never know that they have conceived, let alone that they have miscarried. More than 25 per cent of women miscarry in the first trimester. Approximately one in 200 couples will experience two or more consecutive miscarriages.

According to Professor Lesley Regan, who runs the UK's biggest miscarriage research programme in the UK, there is no single cause for recurrent miscarriages. The five main reasons are:

1. genetic causes
2. hormonal causes
3. blood-clotting disorders
4. infection
5. structural abnormalities of the womb and cervix.

Interestingly, one aspect of the care given at Professor Regan's clinic – which has improved the outcome for women who miscarry, especially for those where there is no known reason for miscarriage – is tender loving care. TLC, as it is often referred to, has been shown to improve outcomes in women who have had access to the supportive staff at their clinic. It is also something that can be easily replicated elsewhere, and demonstrates the mind/body link.

Let's take a closer look at the five main reasons women miscarry.

What Causes Miscarriage?

Genetic Causes

The most common cause for a single miscarriage is a chromosomal abnormality in the developing foetus which makes it incompatible with life. This cause of miscarriage is generally completely random, and is rarely behind recurrent miscarriages. A genetic cause behind recurrent miscarriages affects between 3 and 5 per cent of couples. In these cases there will be an abnormal chromosome pattern present in one parent, repeatedly passed on to the foetus. If this does turn out to be the reason, referral to a clinical geneticist is necessary to determine the specific type of chromosomal abnormality, and whether or not anything can be done about it.

Hormonal Causes

The main hormonal problems that can result in miscarriage:
1. low levels of progesterone
2. polycystic ovary syndrome (PCOS)

Low Levels of Progesterone

Low levels of progesterone, found in women who miscarry, usually arise because of a failure of the egg to implant successfully, which is a trigger for further progesterone production. A good supply of progesterone is necessary to keep the lining of the womb, in which the fertilized egg needs to implant, intact so that pregnancy can continue. Improving a woman's general health, and ensuring that the lining of the womb is well nourished before fertilization, helps create a better environment for implantation.

PCOS

When given a pelvic ultrasound, many women who frequently miscarry are found to have polycystic ovaries. PCOS is a common condition, found in 25 per cent of all women, but not every woman with it will have problems with conception. However, for some there are associated hormonal imbalances, such as raised LH (luteinizing hormone) or testosterone levels. Studies carried out at Professor Regan's clinic have shown that neither PCOS nor a raised LH level is associated with recurrent miscarriage.

Blood-clotting Disorders

Women with abnormal blood-clotting may carry the genes for inherited thrombophilias. Homocysteine builds up in the bloodstream, causing blood clots and hardening of the arteries. It has been known for some time that a woman's blood thickens during pregnancy, but in some women this is more pronounced than others, and can cause little blood clots to occur in the developing placenta. A placenta that is unable to supply the growing foetus with the oxygen and nutrients it needs can lead to miscarriage, premature birth or a 'small for dates' baby (that is, an infant who weighs less than the normal for its age, in the womb or at birth). Testing for the presence of antiphospholipid antibodies (see page 271), which cause the blood to clot more easily than it should, can identify women at risk. Where this risk goes unidentified, and no treatment is given, the miscarriage rate can be up to 90 per cent. However, if identified and treated (by a combination of aspirin and heparin therapy), outcomes are good – up to 70 per cent of women have a chance of successful pregnancy at Professor Regan's clinic treated with combined therapy, and 40 per cent when treated with aspirin alone. I also believe in the benefits of a good diet on blood health – see Nutrition chapter page 108.

Infection

Professor Regan's clinic has identified the role of infection in recurrent miscarriages, and in particular its link to late miscarriage (after 14 weeks' pregnancy). It is less likely to be a risk factor in cases of early recurrent miscarriage.

Screening for infections in both partners is an important part of any infertility and miscarriage investigation. However, infections that can cause a fever (a rise in temperature to over 40 degrees), for example the flu, can put a pregnancy at risk. In any event, any acute or low-grade infection makes a demand on the body's resources, and should be treated not just with the appropriate medical intervention, but also with rest, good nutrition and supplementation.

For more about the infections that can affect your fertility, see the Fertility Work-up chapter.

Structural Abnormalities

The advent of three-dimensional ultrasound scans has made the diagnosis of abnormalities of the womb (such as a uterine septum) more possible. These scans are very similar to the routine, internal ultrasound scans many women are familiar with. Research is currently looking at how common a feature structural abnormalities are in cases of recurrent miscarriage, and whether or not surgical correction improves the outcome.

Cervical incompetence, where the cervix fails to remain closed during pregnancy, only affects pregnancies of longer than 14 weeks. There is no way of knowing whether this will happen, but if it has happened in previous pregnancies a 'purse-string' stitch can be placed at 12 weeks to keep the cervix closed until near the time you are due.

Other Factors

Smoking

There is some evidence to show that smoking increases the risk of miscarriage, and this is related to the number of cigarettes smoked. While five cigarettes a day will probably do little harm, a 40-cigarettes-a-day habit undoubtedly will. In any event, smoking cigarettes also depletes the body of essential B and C vitamins, and makes levels of carbon monoxide rise in the blood, reducing the oxygen content. Smoking also introduces other noxious gases, nicotine and tar to the lungs and bloodstream. Men who smoke are damaging their sperm. So the recommendation for your health, the health of your unborn child and your future children's health, is always to stop!

Alcohol

Women who regularly drink alcohol in excess are also at increased risk of miscarriage. Not only are large quantities of alcohol toxic to the body, placing stress on the liver and kidneys, vital nutrients are often sapped from the body to compensate. The occasional glass of wine probably won't hurt, but an excess and high level of spirits will, so many women choose to give up alcohol completely while trying to conceive. For women who have experienced miscarriage, this is good advice.

VDUs

In the past, there was some concern about women being exposed to VDUs (video display units) from working at computers in early pregnancy. Recent research, however, has shown no association between VDU exposure and miscarriage. It's worth bearing in mind, though, that sitting for long periods doing a repetitive task can be draining on the body. Try and take regular breaks to move around, which will improve blood circulation. Also try to get some fresh air every day, and also to relax and destress with some gentle exercise.

Summary

What might cause a miscarriage?

- Structural abnormalities (such as distortion of the uterine cavity or adhesions caused by surgery or infection) are responsible for 5 to 10 per cent of miscarriages.
- Luteal phase defects (resulting in low progesterone) are responsible for around 20 per cent of miscarriages.
- Genetic (chromosomal) abnormalities are responsible for 5 per cent of miscarriages in women who have never given birth and 50 per cent in women who have already had a baby.

- Immune system abnormalities are responsible for a large percentage of miscarriages (see page 269).
- Infections (bacterial, viral, fungal, parasitic and sexually transmitted) are responsible for around 1 per cent of miscarriages.
- Unknown causes are responsible for around 15 per cent of miscarriages.
- Other possible causes include endocrine or hormonal disorders (such as poorly controlled diabetes, hyperthyroidism or hypothyroidism) and conception factors (such as defective sperm cells, time of egg implantation or stress).

What Are the Risk Factors?

What we can evaluate from previous research are those women most at risk of miscarriage. This includes:

- women who have a previous spontaneous abortion
- being over 35
- having anorexia
- smoking
- having more than two alcoholic drinks a day
- drinking coffee – caffeine stays in a pregnant woman's body much longer than in non-pregnant women. A study of 3,135 pregnant women showed that moderate to heavy caffeine drinkers were more likely to have late-first or second trimester spontaneous abortions than those who didn't drink coffee
- using cocaine
- exposure to X-rays or who spend long periods in aeroplanes
- exposure to excessive amounts of environmental toxins such as lead, mercury or organic solvents

- having a serious illness
- increased levels of homocysteine (which can damage arteries and interfere with the clotting mechanism of the blood).

Treatment

- Surgery may correct most structural defects, although, as mentioned, research is still ongoing.
- Progesterone may be prescribed for the first 12 weeks of pregnancy. Progesterone is responsible for preventing the endometrium (the rich, blood-filled lining of the womb that sustains the growing embryo and foetus) from breaking down.
- Antiphospholipid antibodies (see page 271) can be treated with a low-dose (75-mg) aspirin and/or heparin. Treatment may be most effective if started before conception and continued throughout the pregnancy.
- Anti-nuclear antibodies (which can cause Systemic Lupus Erythematosus – see page 271) can be treated with Prednisolone, a corticosteroid that suppresses the inflammatory process and stabilizes cell processes.
- Immune system abnormalities can be treated with a range of medications.
- Women with abnormal blood-clotting can be treated with low-dose aspirin plus low-molecular-weight heparin injections, beginning before pregnancy occurs and continuing to up to 4 to 6 weeks after birth.

Some of the drug treatments mentioned are highly controversial and would not be recommended by doctors.

Can Complementary Therapies Help?

In my practice I use Traditional Chinese Medicine and acupuncture. Acupuncture works in a number of ways, helping the body repair itself, balancing hormones, reducing stress and improving the blood flow to the pelvic area and womb, thereby providing good incubation for a growing foetus.

As well as addressing the physical considerations, with miscarriage there is a whole range of emotions to deal with. Feelings of guilt, depression, failure, separation, loss, envy and rage are all very common. Being around other women who have babies can be hard. Losing a baby can be especially difficult if you have previously had fertility problems or have miscarried before. You need to be able to work through your feelings at your own pace and with the right support. Counselling, therapy or the right support group can be helpful. Don't bottle up your feelings; do seek this kind of support to help you come through this difficult time.

In my practice, I work with a hypnotherapist. Hypnotherapy (see page 206) can be very effective at counteracting the sort of complex negative and guilty feelings that miscarriage can provoke. It also enables people to reach deep levels of relaxation, manage stress and control the sort of anxiety that can contribute to low levels of depression. Alleviating these feelings helps a woman to feel more focused and centred, and better able to manage the distressing feelings that miscarriage can arouse.

Although not strictly complementary, improving a couple's nutritional status pays dividends when helping avoid recurrent miscarriages. Not only will an improved nutritional status improve the quality of a man's sperm, it can also help with the production and balance of female hormones, and create a better internal environment in which a growing pregnancy can thrive.

I believe that what we eat and how we eat it plays an enormous role in fertility, and although many couples can get away with inadequate nutrition and still manage to get pregnant, for others it is essential to address this issue. The chapter on nutrition (see page 89) is comprehensive on the subject, but there are some specific nutritional deficiencies that relate to miscarriage:

- Low levels of magnesium. Oxidation, a process that is damaging to cell membranes, can lead to loss of magnesium. The recommended dose is 300 to 400 mg a day.
- The antioxidant selenium protects the cell membrane, helping to maintain appropriate levels of magnesium. Women who miscarry have lower levels of selenium than women who carry their babies to full term. The recommended dose is 200 mcg a day.
- Studies suggest levels of Co-enzyme Q10 are lower in women who have had a recent miscarriage. Production of CoQ10 in the body also depends on adequate levels of folic acid, vitamin B_{12} and betaine.
- Vitamins A, E and beta-carotene tend to be lower in women who have miscarried. A good prenatal multi-vitamin will generally supply adequate levels.
- Deficiency of vitamins B_6, B_{12} and folic acid can aggravate levels of homocysteine.

The Implications for Infertility

Too often, couples who miscarry are advised to 'just keep trying', especially if they have already had one successful pregnancy. New studies of immunology, however, show that if a miscarriage is caused by an auto-immune problem, subsequent pregnancies will only make the condition worse. If you are a woman aged over 35, I would recommend that you push your doctor for further testing after a miscarriage. A lot of women can come to feel that their bodies have let them down some-how, while others feel very anxious about trying again because they fear going through another miscarriage. Some couples stay close, while for others a certain distance can set in. Talk things through – with your partner, understanding friends or family members or a trained counsel-lor – and try to remember to look after yourself and your relationship.

assisted conception

Treatment Options

There are many treatment options available to couples today, and the choice you make will depend on your unique circumstances including your age, the results of your blood tests and the various outcomes as your treatment progresses. The most important factor helping you to make a decision is that you both feel you have 'ticked all of the boxes' – have done everything possible and that you are ready to move on to considering assisted conception. I'd recommend that the first step in this process would be to take another look at the 'Crucial Questions' section in the chapter called The Way I Work (page xv).

Having had a variety of tests, you and your clinic will now have a clearer idea of how best to proceed. Do not do anything that you feel unhappy about, and keep doing your own research.

Follicular Tracking

For women who have irregular menstrual cycles, the timing of ovulation can be difficult to predict. Ultrasound scans will be done at weekly intervals during your cycle to determine when ovulation is likely to take place; you and your partner can then have sexual intercourse at the appropriate time. In many cases no medication is needed.

Ovulation Induction (OI)

Ovulation induction or stimulation, using tablets, is a way of kick-starting ovulation to give you a chance to conceive naturally. It is the next stage of treatment for women with irregular periods due to inadequate or imbalanced hormones (in other words, when your ovaries and hormonal system are capable of functioning normally, but your system needs help to ovulate regularly and grow follicles to maturity), or if you are not ovulating because of polycystic ovaries (PCOS – see page 263).

To induce ovulation you'll be given a course of clomiphene citrate (brand names Clomid or Serophene). This is taken orally, in tablet form, usually from Day 2 to Day 5 of your cycle, starting with a dose of 50 mg on the second day of your cycle. Dosage may be increased to 100 mg the following month if you have not ovulated, but doses higher than 150 mg are not recommended and can cause side-effects such as hot flushes or tender breasts.

How Clomiphene Works
Clomiphene binds to the oestrogen receptor sites in the brain, fooling your system into thinking that the amount of oestrogen in the blood is too low. This stimulates the hypothalamus to release more of the hormone GnRH, prompting the pituitary to release more LH (luteinizing hormone) and FSH (follicle-stimulating hormone), causing the follicle to start maturing an egg ready for ovulation. It is generally given to women under the age of 35 but can be given to older women as well, although it is less likely to work in older women.

There is some debate about the use of clomiphene. Some women experience headaches and nausea, weight gain and bloating, and in about 15 per cent of women too many follicles develop (this is known as ovarian hyper-stimulation). Regular monitoring is vital; ultrasound scans will check the development and number of follicles in the ovaries. If more than three large follicles have developed, treatment may be suspended because of the increased risk of multiple pregnancy.

Clomiphene will affect the quality of your cervical secretions and the lining of the uterus, and should not be given for more than three cycles without a break. There is some research to show that large doses of vitamin C (1,000 mg a day) will potentiate the action of clomiphene. You must have a break for a month after taking Clomid for three months. There are some concerns that women who have undergone ovarian stimulation may be at an increased risk of ovarian cancer later in life, therefore it is important not to take Clomid continuously for a long period of time. Discuss this with your doctor and devise a treatment plan that will be suitable for you.

Figures show that after a course of clomiphene, around 80 per cent of women with irregular or no ovulation will ovulate and around 50 per cent will conceive, the majority of them within three months. Women over the age of 40, however, do not seem to respond well to the drug.

For a lot of women, clomiphene treatment is a gentle introduction to assisted conception techniques, and worth giving a try. Some women sail through a course of treatment, while others experience side-effects such as mood swings and PMT-like symptoms.

Clomiphene and hCG

When ovulation induction using just clomiphene hasn't been successful, the next step may be to give an injection of hCG (human Chorionic Gonadotrophin) to encourage the final maturation of the follicle and release of the egg. It is generally given when one follicle reaches a diameter of at least 18 mm. Sexual intercourse or IUI (see page 305) will be timed for 36 to 40 hours after the hCG injection.

The use of this treatment will depend on a number of factors:
1. There are no blocked tubes.

2. That the sperm are OK.

3. Age – very often, even though this is the first line of treatment, you have to consider that if you are over 38 and have tried this treatment for three to six months you will sometimes be better advised to go straight on to IVF.

IUI – Intra-Uterine Insemination

This may be the next step when ovulation induction using clomiphene alone, or a combination of clomiphene and hCG, hasn't been successful.

The aim of IUI is to place as many active sperm as possible as close as possible to the egg. It is a way of assisting natural fertilization in the womb, and can be valuable when sperm parameters are a little below normal, giving the sperm a kick-start to get nearer to the Fallopian tubes. It is also sometimes used in cases of 'unexplained infertility'.

How IUI Works

After ovulation, a sample of sperm is placed directly into the womb via a catheter (thin tube) passed through the cervix. The procedure is not recommended for women with blocked Fallopian tubes or where there is a more severe problem with sperm count or sperm quality. It generally involves the use of drugs to stimulate the follicles and induce ovulation. According to research, three to four follicles give the best chance of success; any more increases the risk of a multiple pregnancy.

IUI and hMG

With IUI alone, there is a 3 to 6 per cent rate of success per cycle. Clomiphene with IUI increases this to 9 per cent, while hMG (human Menopausal Gonadotrophin, a group of drugs that contain FSH and LH) with IUI increases this to 15 to 20 per cent. This is given to women who haven't responded to Clomid. What this does mean, however, is that you will probably need to have daily injections, to ensure you have a good crop of eggs at ovulation.

Q & As

What is the best timing for IUI?

The procedure is performed as close as possible (ideally within six hours) to the expected time of ovulation, which is determined by an ultrasound scan or by using an ovulation-predictor kit. Ovulation may also be artificially induced with hCG injections. Sometimes two IUIs are scheduled 24 hours apart. Once the egg is fertilized, implantation should take place 6 to 7 days later and the pregnancy should proceed as normal.

How long does it take and is it painful?

The procedure takes only a few minutes and should cause little or no discomfort. Occasionally a little cramping is felt when the catheter is passed through the cervix, and afterwards, but this is probably more to do with ovulation than the IUI. You may also feel wet because the cervix is washed before the catheter is put in. It is best to remain lying down for 15 to 20 minutes after the procedure and then to take it easy for a while. If you have any bleeding, you should abstain from sexual intercourse for 48 hours.

Do I need to rest after having IUI?

Yes. Generally, I feel that clinics don't allow you long enough after the procedure for this. IUI can be, for some women, quite a cold, clinical procedure, and I recommend that you go straight home and put your feet up or go to bed. Certainly give yourself the rest of the day off work. The sperm cannot fall out, as some women imagine, but you want to do everything in your power to ensure the procedure is successful. You should not go swimming for 7 days after an IUI. Sex, on the other hand, is recommended after an initial 48-hour lapse!

When should the sperm be collected?

A sperm sample needs to be with the clinic within 30 minutes of ejaculation into a sterile container. The sample must be taken not fewer than 2 days nor more than 5 days after the male's previous ejaculation. The sample is then 'washed' to separate sperm from semen and motile sperm from non-motile sperm, a process which can take up to 2 hours. Most clinics perform the IUI as soon as the sperm are prepared, though washed sperm can remain potent for up to 24 hours.

What if my partner is unable to produce sperm of an adequate quality?

You have the option of using donated sperm. All sperm donors are tested for HIV, hepatitis, cystic fibrosis and blood group, and screened very carefully to take into account medical and family history. Sperm are then quarantined for six months and re-tested. Specific counselling will be given to explore all the implications of such treatment. Sperm donation is *only* for those cases when absolutely no sperm are produced in the testes or if the sperm carry a genetic defect that will affect the foetus.

How many IUIs should we try before moving on to IVF?

This is a difficult question to answer. Generally you should look at trying this for four to six months (as a general rule, three to four IUIs using Clomid, followed by three to four attempts with injections, should bring success). If you are over 38, keep an eye on your fertility) and FSH (see page 251). If you have not met with success after several treatments, you might want to consider moving on to IVF.

Moving On to IVF

Once the decision has been made and the clinic chosen, generally couples feel relieved that they are being proactive. I find that many of the couples we plan IVF for actually get pregnant naturally in the interim – it's as if they have let go of something.

Remember, as a woman it is not only your decision but your partner's, also. Disagreements about starting IVF are very common. A woman may go ahead and do all the research, then come home and make an announcement: 'We're starting.' Very often her partner is not ready and doesn't understand the process. Reaching a deadlock over this just adds to both partners' stress levels.

Women learn fast; sometimes it takes men longer to catch up. Don't feel that your partner is blocking your chance of getting pregnant by not going along with what you want. Be patient and try to reach a decision together. The positive side of this is that it makes you both stop and think and understand things from each other's perspective.

This can also be an issue after one course of IVF has failed. Very often women are keen to start again as soon as possible, while their partners are not so sure. Again, be patient with each other and try to understand your partner's point of view.

I believe passionately in the importance of preparing for IVF. There is a great deal that can be done to support a couple, increasing their chance of a positive outcome with assisted conception, and success rates are improving all the time.

Nowadays, with so much information available to couples via books, websites and Internet chat rooms, many have a pretty clear idea of what assisted conception involves. They also have their own ideas about what to expect and, often, misconceptions about what is possible in their case. Many couples feel, often wrongly, that assisted conception is the only course of action open to them after having failed to get pregnant naturally immediately. My role is to find out about their personal situation, diagnosis or problems, and define a course of action that is specific to them, based on their own particular circumstances.

The decision to undergo IVF is, of course, a big one to take. Embarking on IVF comes with physical, mental, emotional and financial costs that need to be weighed up. At our clinic we encourage women to feel very positive about it, because if you feel supported and understand the process this can be a great help before, during and after treatment. IVF has come a long way, and the science is being perfected all the time. By going to a clinic with a good track record and cutting-edge treatments, couples are now very often conceiving within a couple of cycles. And with the advent of the Internet, women in particular are doing more and more of their own research about the clinics they should attend. Many are travelling overseas. I feel very sad when I see couples who have gone through numerous IVF attempts at clinics where they really haven't received a good service. Some feel they have reached the end of the road because they believe that IVF is just the one technique. This is not the case. Many of my clients start out by going (via a GP referral) to a clinic, then realize by looking around that other clinics do things differently. The way that you are stimulated, the amount of monitoring (scans, blood tests, etc.) that is done – all have an impact on the chances of success. Many couples stay in a comfort zone, remaining loyal to a clinic where they like the nurses or the convenient travelling time to get there. But loyalty is a luxury couples cannot afford: sometimes you have to move out of your comfort zone and change clinics if the one you're at isn't working for you, or they're not changing the treatments they offer you with each attempt. Maybe you should consider moving on.

Even after 30 years, IVF is still an imperfect procedure and the results vary widely, depending on the reasons it has been recommended.

I would advise all couples to think seriously about their general health and fertility before they embark on IVF. While IVF is a technique designed to create one or more fertilized eggs, it is only part of the process. Conception requires good specimens of egg and sperm to start with, successful implantation into an enriched womb lining, and a good supply of balanced hormones to continue the pregnancy to term.

I believe that you have to prepare for IVF just as you would for a natural pregnancy. The research shows that stress, weight and even the time of year can influence the success rate of IVF (with the winter months seeing a drop in this). Laying down good ground work is vitally important. I also believe hugely in working with orthodox Western medicine alongside supporting treatments during an IVF cycle.

I believe strongly that, as far as possible, it is best to work in harmony with nature. In my experience (and this is backed up by research), IVF works better in spring, summer and the time for growth and renewal within nature's cycle. In winter, nature is dormant and the body naturally needs to conserve energy and rest.

It is also worth saying that, even though most people automatically think of IVF when they think of assisted reproductive technologies, there are, in fact, a number of different forms of assisted conception, of which IVF is just one. These include not just the methods already discussed (ovulation-stimulating drugs like clomiphene, IUI) but also artificial insemination (which may utilize a partner's sperm or donor sperm) and egg donation. Then, within IVF, there are different approaches such as ICSI (intra-cytoplasmic sperm injection), where sperm are actually injected into the egg. To be able to undergo IVF, the female needs functioning ovaries and some male sperm. There's more about this later in this chapter.

Preparation Programme

At our clinic, because I believe so deeply that preparation for IVF can help the outcome, I have devised a programme specifically to improve a couple's chances of conceiving and carrying a healthy baby to term. Much of this programme is the same as for preparing to conceive normally – focusing on good nutrition, detox, stress management and relaxation – because these things are just as relevant, if not more so, for couples undergoing assisted conception.

Detox, in particular, is important for women who have already had numerous IVF cycles and are suffering from the after-effects of heavy doses of powerful drugs (some women put on weight as a result of the drugs, for example). The liver in particular will have been working overtime. Although women will have to go through cycles of drugs again, it is still well worth reducing your toxic load and strengthening your body, mind and spirit beforehand.

There is also considerable research to show the extent to which stress affects IVF outcomes. This is hardly surprising, and is why I emphasize that clients learn and practise stress-management techniques – breathing exercises, relaxation, visualization and meditation (see page 184), and also hypnotherapy when necessary. Stress has an adverse affect on the fertility hormones, and given that your body will be coping with hormonal therapy to suppress ovulation and then stimulate the ovaries, reducing stress helps to relax you and gives you techniques that will help you cope with what you're going through.

I always recommend that a programme to support the body – for both women and men – begins two to three months before a new IVF cycle, with a detox (see page 141). For women, especially where there have been previous, unsuccessful cycles of assisted conception, I will also recommend MLD (manual lymphatic drainage), abdominal massage and acupuncture. Acupuncture starts a week before a new IVF cycle is due to begin, and is given regularly throughout the IVF cycle. We use electro-acupuncture to enhance the use of the needles to help in the growth of follicles and building up the womb lining between egg collection and transfer. This is especially important to stimulate pelvic blood flow, ensuring that the womb is well prepared for implantation when the embryos are transferred.

Preparing for IVF

IVF is a very hi-tech procedure. Many women worry so much about starting IVF; it can feel like a huge leap into the unknown. IVF requires drugs that change the function of the body's hormonal system, and it is understandable that many women will be very worried about possible side-effects. I can certainly understand why many women get so concerned about the drugs they have to put into their bodies during the course of IVF. You feel that you are doing everything naturally to prepare, then just adding drugs to your system – it can feel wrong, as if you are flying in the face of your body's instincts.

If you have opted for the IVF route, try to view the drugs as just part of the process that will help you reach your goal: having a baby. There is also a great deal that you can do to help the outcome and to give yourself a greater sense of control over the course of events. A lot of fear and anxiety can be alleviated by having a good understanding of how IVF uses the body's own processes, the particular objectives of treatments and the possible results. This knowledge can help you to strengthen your own natural resources and visualize a successful outcome. Everyone comes to IVF from a different perspective, with different emotional, physical and psychological issues, yet very many women feel, once they have started, that it is never as bad as they'd anticipated. Often it is the *thought* of treatment looming that is the hardest part to deal with.

1. Research – It is important to get the right treatment from the beginning, because your chances of success are best the first and second time you have IVF. As your body starts to get used to the treatment over subsequent attempts, your response may decline.

2. Move out of your comfort zone – Just because your clinic is near your work, it isn't necessarily the best one for you.

3. Time – Look at your life and work schedule and make sure you won't be over-stressing yourself. You need to build in at least seven hours a week for appointments, scans, blood tests, etc. Many IVF clinics are incredibly busy and don't always run to time. In addition, build in time to give yourself treats and enough rest throughout the process.

4. Support – Make sure you have a supportive partner or friend whom you can chat to as you go through the process.

5. Build up your reserves prior to starting treatment: sleep, meditate and exercise, to help you feel good about starting the process. And you do need to view it is as process – don't limit yourselves to thinking 'We're only doing this once'. Often the first time gives a clinic a good indication of how you respond to the drugs and how it's going to work for you.

6. Be positive – But keep your feet firmly on the ground. Don't set yourself time limits, and be prepared to move the goalposts if circumstances change – as very often they will!

7. Keep having sex prior to starting IVF – I give couples who come to our clinic a four- to six-month window to try and conceive naturally before embarking on IVF – and so many of them become pregnant before the treatment starts. Many couples think 'We're doing IVF so we don't have to have sex anymore.' This kind of thinking could damage your relationship and will place unnecessary restrictions on your chances of conceiving naturally. However, once you are undergoing IVF treatment you should not have sex.

Visualization

As suggested in the chapter called Thoughts and Emotions (page 192), while preparing for IVF (and as you go through each stage of treatment) it's good to visualize what is happening and what you want to happen in your body – the eggs maturing, the womb lining ripening, the embryos implanting (many clinics will have images of the process to help you to visualize this). The temptation for many couples is to put what's happening out of their minds, but I suggest daily positive affirmations. To these you can add some statements about how well your body is responding to and processing the drugs. You may feel a little silly doing this, but the mind is an incredibly powerful tool. Believe that you ARE going to have a baby and that in the course of treatment you ARE going to remain healthy and not compromise your body's natural defence mechanisms or immune system. I am convinced that a positive mindset can make all the difference. Equally I know it can be hard, particularly as time goes on and you've had a couple of failed attempts, but stick with it.

Nutrition

Good diet and nutrition are vital in preparation for IVF to support your body's ability for:
- developing and growing eggs
- building the lining of the womb
- helping with healing after retrieval of the eggs
- and for the implantation of the embryo following transfer.

Your diet should concentrate on building up those body systems that are going to come under most stress during the IVF process.

The liver is the major detoxifying organ, helping to get rid of drugs and toxins. Almost two quarts of blood pass through the liver every minute. Cleansing the liver prior to treatment, especially if you have already been through a cycle of IVF drugs, can be very helpful. Certain nutrients and vitamins help to optimize liver function, protect it from toxins and increase the rate at which it excretes toxins (see page 156).

- When the liver metabolizes toxins, free radicals are produced which need to be neutralized by antioxidants such as vitamin C, vitamin E, selenium, bioflavanoids and glutathione (an amino acid) – all essential for protecting the liver. I put my clients on a multi-vitamin and -mineral.

- EFAs (essential fatty acids), which are very good for the cell membranes. I particularly recommend DHA.

- Silymarin is the most potent liver-protective agent, helping to regenerate new liver cells. Take a silymarin supplement three times a day and eat plenty of seeds, fruits and green leaves.

All of these nutrients – and the ones mentioned later in this section – can be taken in the two to three months leading up to starting IVF. It is better, where possible, to have a nutritional consultation. In addition, follow the guidelines outlined in the Nutrition chapter (beginning on page 89).

The question of egg quality will become one of your overriding concerns during the course of your treatment. Animal studies have shown that insufficient protein in your diet can result in a reduced number of eggs. Make sure you have an adequate supply of protein. Protein is the major functional and structural component of all the cells in the body. Our enzymes, hormones, immune cells and blood-clotting molecules as well as the skin, muscle, hair and nails are made of protein, and during periods of extra growth and development it is especially important to ensure adequate amounts of protein in the diet. In order to allow for the extra demands of producing several healthy, well-nourished eggs, the protein needs of a woman embarking on IVF are slightly higher than normal – around 55g a day.

I see so many women on high-protein diets; these can be detrimental, although it has to be said that you would have to be eating really large quantities to experience negative effects. Vegetarians – and particularly vegans – have to be extra-vigilant to ensure they're eating a wide variety of foods, which should include pulses, nuts and seeds, to ensure they're getting all the amino acids they need.

Milk

In some clinics, women are often asked to drink large quantities of milk to prepare for IVF. This is because milk is a 'complete protein' containing a composition of amino acids similar to that found in human body protein. Thus, if you are drinking a litre of milk a day your clinic can be absolutely sure you are having adequate protein. However, if your diet is generally healthy and varied it should be quite possible to get adequate amounts of protein without having to drink this much milk.

Soya

While soya is a good source of protein, particularly for vegetarians, I do not advise that you consume soya milk as a substitute for cow's milk, nor that you consume whole soya beans. Soya products such as tofu, miso, tamari and tempeh should be restricted to three times a week. This is because soya contains hormone-like substances called phytoestrogens and research to date has been inconclusive as to the effect of these plant oestrogens on fertility generally and on hormone-suppressing and -stimulating drugs (like those taken during IVF treatment) in particular.

The best-quality protein foods, in terms of amino acid balance, include eggs, meat, fish, beans, lentils and quinoa. Opt for organic meat where you can, and avoid too many dairy products – get your protein from other sources. For ideas on protein meal plans, see page 123 in the Nutrition chapter.

EFAs (essential fatty acids) are vitally important, not least because most of us are deficient in them. Omega-3 fatty acids, of which DHA is one, are especially important for hormone balance. My recommendation is for a DHA supplement in the lead-up to IVF treatment, then doubling the amount you take during treatment.

If you have been trying to conceive, you and your partner may already be taking supplements. If not, invest in the best-quality preconception multi-vitamins and -minerals you can afford, and start taking them at least three to four months before IVF treatment commences. Studies have shown that where women take a supplement, the fluid which surrounds and nourishes the eggs is rich in vitamins C and E. Zinc, magnesium and vitamin A are all vital for egg production, and selenium and magnesium have been shown to improve fertilization rates. Make sure that your vitamin A intake doesn't exceed the RDA (recommended daily allowance) as it is fat soluble, so isn't excreted, and you want to avoid a build-up in the body prior to pregnancy – vitamin A in high doses has been linked with foetal disorders.

Other vitamins to be considered include:

Vitamin B_1 is vital for enriching your womb lining in preparation for implantation. Vitamin B_6 (a necessary precursor for progesterone), iron and CoQ10 are all wonderful for ensuring a good flow of oxygen around the body, which supports cell metabolism. (See also Nutrition chapter, beginning on page 89.)

Egg retrieval and the other invasive procedures you will undergo are regarded as minor surgery, but you need to be able to repair quickly to receive the incoming embryos. Take vitamin C (1,000 mg) and zinc (20 mg) daily for at least two weeks beforehand, and the homoeopathic remedy *arnica 6c* four times a day from the day before the procedure.

Checklist

- A multivitamin and -mineral and EFAs.
- Vitamin C will help collagen production and is vital for wound-healing following egg retrieval (there is also evidence suggesting it can help to prevent miscarriage).
- Vitamin E enhances healing.
- A good intake of B vitamins will help your body cope with stress.
- Make sure your diet contains sufficient zinc. Zinc promotes cell-formation and wound-healing after any form of surgery and is vital for hormone production and implantation. Many of the women who come to see me with fertility problems are zinc deficient.
- A healthy overall diet, especially if you have detoxed, makes sense. Avoid chocolate, sugary foods, salty snacks, coffee, tea, cola, all fizzy drinks and alcohol. They rob your body of vital nutrients and have a diuretic effect. Also avoid processed foods.
- If you have already been through one cycle of IVF, give yourself a break of a month or two to allow your ovaries to recover.
- You give IVF a better chance of working if you are not over weight. If you are, sort out your eating habits so that you can lose weight slowly and gradually, without robbing yourself of vital nutrients. Likewise, if you are seriously underweight, look at your diet to help you gain the weight you need sensibly.
- Do not smoke and avoid smoky atmospheres. Smoking affects fertility.

- Drink a minimum of 2 litres of water (filtered or bottled still) a day. This is in addition to other fluids you consume in the day, including herbal teas. One of the effects of dehydration is to switch off the thirst signal in the brain. It is no good starting to drink just before you begin procedures – that would be like pouring water onto a parched plant: the water will run straight out the bottom of the pot without being absorbed. The body needs time to become properly hydrated.
- Try to avoid aerobic exercise while going through a cycle of IVF (though in the months leading up to treatment, exercise is fine). Instead, take gentle exercise such as walking or yoga.
- If you have any recurrent bladder or kidney infections, get these sorted out first – any infection depletes the body's immune system and makes extra nutritional demands.

Complementary Therapies

There are many complementary therapies that may help while you are planning or going through IVF. Don't go and do hundreds of treatments, however – plan a course that suits you after taking a look at areas of weakness in your life and how stressed you are, then you can make an informed choice from among the many options such as acupuncture, hypnotherapy, massage, reflexology, etc. And keep in mind that good nutrition (see Nutrition chapter beginning on page 89) can be a kind of medicine in itself!

Acupuncture can be highly beneficial in preparation for IVF, during the treatment cycle and to rebalance the body following a failed cycle. Acupuncture on a weekly basis helps to detoxify and balance the body, build up the womb lining, grow follicles and, post-transfer, will help with implantation and maintaining pregnancy. In Chinese medicine, the liver is associated with anger, frustration and irritability, emotions that women often complain of when they are on IVF drugs. The Chinese theory is that acupuncture at certain key points on the liver meridian helps you to feel more calm and less irritable.

In Traditional Chinese Medicine the kidneys are considered to play a vital role in reproduction. Kidney energy gets weaker as we age, with deficiency often showing up as lower backache around menstruation or a weakness behind the knees. Certain acupuncture points are believed in Chinese medicine to build up the kidney energies, increasing the chance of conception and reducing the risk of miscarriage.

If acupuncture is not an option for you, try at least to keep your lower back and lower abdomen warm in the lead-up to egg collection, using a hot water bottle. This 'lower *chou*' area, between the umbilicus and the pubic bone, is regarded as crucially important for conception and pregnancy and has many important acupuncture points. I find many women are very cold in this area; I encourage them to keep it warm.

Rest between 5 and 7 p.m., the most important part of the day for kidney function according to Chinese medicine. Put your feet up for a bit if you can at this time of day.

Reflexology can be helpful in preparation for IVF, particularly on the parts of the foot corresponding to the pelvis and lymphatic system. Be sure to tell a reflexologist that you are planning a pregnancy.

If you have suffered from any back injuries or problems in the past, I recommend a course of chiropractic or osteopathy.

Explore relaxation techniques to find one that suits you and fits into your life easily. Try hypnotherapy, meditation, yoga, tai chi.

Starting IVF Treatment

I think it is so important to feel positive that you have ticked all the boxes and are ready to go before you start IVF treatment, because you are embarking on a bit of a roller-coaster ride and you need to do so with confidence. It may be a bit bewildering at first, but you will quickly pick up the terminology used and learn about the protocols and treatments offered at your clinic. Most, however, offer two treatment protocols: a long protocol and a short protocol (see below). Having said this, as we learn more and more, procedures and protocols are changing all the time.

Once a woman has decided to move on to IVF she is generally relieved, but sometimes she can't get past the first hurdle because, out of the blue, her hormones (particularly follicle-stimulating hormone, or FSH – see page 251) may have gone up. This can leave you feeling cheated or even quite devastated. Different clinics have different protocols for the FSH level required: some believe that it should be below 10 before treatment is started, others do not go by this rule. Some women whose FSH is raised or high feel very optimistic about getting their levels down by using complementary therapies such as the herbal remedy agnus castus or acupuncture. Be wary of practitioners or therapists who don't help things by giving you false expectations, sometimes getting women to wait months before trying IVF when age and fertility are not on their side. Age has a big part to play in the significance of FSH levels and their relevance. High FSH levels are indicative that fertility is waning and sometimes, even if they do come down, this doesn't mean that an IVF treatment will succeed. Many of these women have a greater success with egg donation. Some women will have a go at IVF regardless, feeling that it might just work. This is a decision that you and your partner have to make for yourselves, and certainly sometimes it does work.

The worst thing for women with raised FSH levels is hearing the word 'menopausal'. It completely freaks most women out and often the way the news is delivered is brutal: 'The only option left is egg donation.' Very often this will be the first time a woman has heard the word 'menopausal' used about herself and she is not ready to hear it. She is shocked and feels that she is on the scrap heap. The word 'menopausal' makes a lot of women feel that they are about to turn, overnight, into a frazzled dried-up prune.

FSH levels are important, and yes, if they are high this is not a good sign, but I honestly believe at looking at the whole picture – stress levels, lifestyle, nutrition and giving women a bit of breathing space – to see if a 'fertility window' can be created one month where levels are good enough to commence IVF or even get pregnant naturally. I have seen all sorts of things happen – women who conceive naturally, women whose levels have come right down and go on to succeed with IVF, and, also, women who have come to accept that egg donation is the route for them.

IVF Challenges Every Relationship
I tell all of my patients – you will have good and bad days. There will always be a low point in the cycle when you feel tearful and upset. It could be that you have been for a scan and been told that you haven't got many follicles, only to go back next day and be told that everything is fine. You may also find yourself feeling frustrated with the clinic if it seems they are not taking enough time over you or giving you enough support. All of these feelings are normal. There are so many hurdles to get through; you have to accept this from the start.

Couples start out down this route on an equal footing, visiting the doctor together at the same level of understanding. Women move on very fast, leaving their men behind very quickly. Within two weeks a woman will know all the technical details of IVF and how it works –

just don't expect your man to be the same. It is not that he isn't interested or doesn't care, it's just that it doesn't mean the same thing to him.
I have seen so many women get upset during an IVF cycle because their
partner wasn't over the moon when they came back from a scan to tell
him they had eight follicles and a womb lining of 8.5 centimetres. These
details become so important to women – seven follicles rather than
eight, the size of the follicles, etc. – but if you give your partner a hard
time because he isn't up to speed on the significance of all this, no one
benefits.

Your relationship is so important. If you have a bad day – maybe the
news from a scan hasn't been that good, or you haven't been able to get
through to the clinic or are just feeling angry, tearful, frustrated – don't
take it out on your partner. I advise all of my clients to spend 10 minutes at the end of each day talking over what you are feeling and really
trying to see it from each other's point of view.

The process of IVF, and in particular the high doses of hormones a
woman has to tolerate, affects her physically and emotionally, and can
put an enormous strain not just on her but on her relationship. She may
feel resentful sometimes that she is going through so much while her
partner's life carries on almost as usual. He, for his part, may be feeling
very guilty about all she is going through. There may also be anxieties
about the financial costs (only a relatively small provision is made for
IVF by the NHS). And there is often the extra burden of expectations
and pressure from your own parents and other family members. Any
relationship that manages to cope with all this is very strong, and that
is an achievement in itself that should be celebrated.

The Long Protocol

A protocol is a set of guidelines regarding what a clinic will do during
an IVF cycle – injections, scans, blood tests, removal of eggs and egg

transfer. These guidelines are not set in stone and will vary according to your individual circumstances. For example, some clinics may start you on the Pill prior to IVF treatment.

The long protocol starts on Day 21 of your cycle. You will be given suppression drugs to sniff, to down-regulate your cycle. This is done in order to dampen down the ovaries and stop any follicles developing. It enables the doctors to start with a 'clean slate', so to speak, so that when you get your period you can be given injections as well, in the hope of producing lots of eggs.

Understandably, many women are nervous about the drugs they need to sniff, and symptoms such as headaches are common. Flu-like symptoms and dizziness can also sometimes occur. Many women feel emotionally fragile – is it any wonder when your system has been shut down?

Tips for Coping

- Give in to this feeling.
- Go to bed early, drink plenty of water, take a good multivitamin and DHA.
- Don't force your body to go to the gym, run or exercise – work with what your body is going through. Rest is so important, all the energy you have, no matter what protocol you are doing, needs to go into the growing of follicles and the building of the womb lining. It is my belief that too much exercise will detract from this.

Possible Hurdles at This Point

Your body may not shut down – you go for a scan and they may find that you have a cyst or a follicle left from a previous cycle. This will mean that you will be on the medication for longer.

You may not bleed; in this case drugs may be given to make you bleed. This can be quite demoralizing and add to your stress levels, and also prolongs the length of time you will require treatment. I usually use acupuncture during down-regulation to help bring on a bleed – certain acupoints below the umbilicus (navel) and on the arms and legs are useful for this purpose.

The Short Protocol

If your hormonal cycle is not stable or regular, you will probably be advised to start assisted conception based on the 'short protocol'. All women on IVF go through this, whether or not they have already gone through a suppression stage (see page 324) first. The short protocol (also known as stimulation or the flare regime) takes advantage of the natural flare-up in FSH (and LH levels) around Day 2 to 3 of your cycle.

After a scan and blood test, you will be given injections morning and evening starting on day 3 or 5 of your cycle. The drug used will depend on your body chemistry and will probably be a combination of LH and FSH, which will fool your ovaries into working overtime to turn out multiple eggs per cycle.

Common brand names include Menogon, Menopure, Puragon, Metrodin High Purity and Gonal-F. Each drug has a slightly different combination of FSH and LH; your doctor will decide which one is suitable for you.

Every woman responds differently, some only needing a small dose and others needing a higher dose to produce the same effect.

You will also continue to take a small amount of the suppression drugs. This will maintain the delicate balance in the body which allows a number of eggs to grow at once and prevents you ovulating before the clinic has a chance to retrieve your eggs.

Your progress will be closely monitored. Ultrasound scans of the ovaries, and blood tests to measure the level of oestradiol, will check how the follicles are developing. Your doctor will also measure the thickness of your womb lining, which needs to be around 10 mm to receive the embryo.

Depending on how your body is responding, the drug dosage will be increased or decreased, within a range of 150 to 450 mg.

When you have a scan, if possible take your partner with you, or at least make sure you can reach him at the end of a phone, as you may well feel the need to talk through the results with him and discuss the implications. He may be able to help you keep a balanced attitude and stop you going into a panic at the slightest less-than-positive word from your doctor. Remember that clinics scan people all of the time. You may find yourself lying there hanging on every word, looking for a reaction or some nugget of information as to how it is all going. You may even start to feel that the doctor or staff are withholding information. Take it from me: If not a lot is said, the chances are it is all going OK! And while any comment such as, 'Not many' might send you into doom-and-gloom mode, remember that the chances are that, though you may have the odd 'bad scan day', you could just as easily go the next day and all will be OK again.

Generally between 10 and 20 follicles will ripen, varying in size from 18 to 23 mm, but at this stage it is impossible to tell if the eggs can be collected from them all. Remember, it is quality, not quantity, that counts when it comes to eggs. On average, around 90 per cent of visible follicles will produce a collectable egg, but a large number of eggs does not necessarily mean that they will all be of good quality. Don't panic and become despondent if you only have five or six. The number of follicles can become so important to women – amounts become crucial and you get angry if your partner can't seem to take this on board. OK, you may only have six, but wait and see what the eggs are like.

Try to stay positive, as hard as it may sometimes seem. Use visualization, drink plenty of water, whatever it takes to keep from giving in to negativity.

Injections

Around day 9, a final scan will check the number and size of eggs, and a blood test will check your level of oestradiol, confirming when to give you an injection (common brand names are Pregnyl and Profasi). This mimics the natural surge of LH which triggers ovulation, encouraging eggs to complete their maturation and causing the follicles to rupture and release the eggs. The eggs are generally retrieved 36 hours later.

Giving Yourself Injections

Your clinic will give you clear guidelines on how to administer injections yourself, but if you are terrified at the very thought, talk to your clinic and GP to find the most practical way to organize having it done under medical supervision. Alternatively, get your partner involved, so long as he's not too squeamish. Many partners overcome their initial nervousness to become expert at injections, and are happy to have a chance to contribute.

Sometimes, following the injection, the area can feel hot. A dab of aloe vera soothes and cools this. As long as the skin isn't broken, you can rub in arnica cream to avoid any bruising. Lastly (and even though this may seem a contradiction in terms), warm up the area by briskly rubbing it or applying warmth from a heating pad or hot water bottle: this brings the blood supply to the surface, making the muscle less tense and more receptive, and resulting in less pain.

Possible Hurdles at This Point

The various hurdles that you need to overcome at this stage include:

- a poor response to the drugs
- Ovarian Hyper-stimulation Syndrome (OHSS – see below)
- problems with your womb lining
- unpleasant side-effects (see below).

Poor Response

About 10 per cent of women do not respond to stimulation, which means oestrogen levels are low and the follicles are not growing. The definition of 'poor response' varies from clinic to clinic. Some clinics test FSH levels at the beginning of the cycle to get an indication of how you will respond. Careful monitoring will allow the drug dosage to be increased or reduced as necessary. If you respond poorly, don't give up hope. A first IVF cycle is very much a case of trial and error, finding out how you will respond and what combinations will suit you best. It is not always possible to get it right first time. Talk to your doctor about varying the drugs for your next cycle or, if you feel it necessary, arrange to move to another clinic.

I am often amazed by the number of women who come to me after having had only one failed cycle, having been told they are poor responders. Very often the way you are stimulated and the drug regime used can make a big difference. In many of these cases I have recommended that the women change clinics, and they have gone on to get pregnant.

Ovarian Hyper-stimulation Syndrome

Some degree of over-stimulation occurs in all women going through this procedure, because the drugs are making the ovaries produce as many eggs, in one go, as they normally would in more than a whole year of ovulation. In order to prevent Ovarian Hyper-stimulation Syndrome (OHSS), careful monitoring is required to ensure you are not growing too many follicles. Women with PCOS (see page 263) are particularly at risk of this happening.

If your doctor is concerned that too many follicles have grown and your oestradiol level is high, you may be left to 'coast'. That means that the hCG injection will be withheld, your stimulation drugs will be stopped and suppression will continue. You will be closely monitored until the level comes down and it is safe to proceed. Bed rest and drinking at least 2 litres of water a day will help at this point.

Occasionally the ovaries get massively enlarged and fluid starts to build up in the abdomen and thorax. Symptoms of OHSS include:

- severe pain in the lower abdomen
- difficulty breathing
- nausea and vomiting
- feeling faint
- reduced urination

In extreme cases OHSS can result in thrombosis, heart attack or stroke. The condition can develop very quickly, which is one of the reasons why regular monitoring at this stage is so important. Make yourself familiar with these symptoms, and if you feel any of them, contact your clinic or hospital immediately.

For some women who have had previous ectopic pregnancies or tubal damage, fluid can build up in the Fallopian tubes. This is toxic, and if it filters into the uterus it will impede implantation. This is known as *hydrosalphinx.* If it happens to you, your doctor will drain the fluid before transfer, or tie off or remove the tube.

Unpleasant Side-effects

On the whole, women do not seem to suffer many side-effects. Some feel tired, but this can be put down to having to stay up late to give yourself injections or to generally feeling emotionally fragile.

Some women, however, do experience unpleasant side-effects which can include:
- abdominal bloating and discomfort
- nausea or diarrhoea
- weight gain
- fever and aching muscles and joints
- tiredness, partly because the timing of injections may interfere with your normal sleep patterns
- headaches caused by hormonal fluctuations
- bruising or rashes at the site of the injection
- mood swings caused by hormonal fluctuations.

Remember, this stage does not last for long. The majority of symptoms will disappear when you have completed the course of injections. But you are, quite literally, at the mercy of your hormones and for a few days will be riding an emotional roller-coaster. This can make you difficult to live with and your partner may find that it is impossible to say or do the right thing. All he can do is to look on helplessly and make irritatingly reassuring comments! Try, both of you, to observe your mood swings objectively instead of getting sucked into them. As I said earlier, try to spend 10 minutes at the end of each day telling one another how you are feeling. Accept each other's support and, if you're feeling bad, just try not to take it out on your partner.

Your Womb Lining

The womb lining should be around 10 mm prior to implantation. Poor womb lining may be the result of a previous infection in the uterus or fibroids. If the womb lining does not thicken up during the stimulation programme, this can be a problem.

Natural tips for thickening the womb lining:

- Take a daily supplement of vitamin E.
- Take a daily supplement of vitamin B_1.
- Eat foods rich in iron such as pumpkin seeds and almonds.
- Include nuts, spinach, seeds, kelp, garlic, kidney beans, milk, brown rice and oatmeal in your diet.
- Eat foods containing bioflavanoids, such as citrus fruits, broccoli, grapes and tomatoes.
- L arginine and amino acid have been shown to increase the womb lining.
- Acupuncture helps with pelvic blood flow and womb lining.
- Keep the lower abdomen warm with the use of a hot water bottle.

Viagra (common brand name Sildena, given orally in this country but by vaginal suppository in the US) may be prescribed to improve blood flow to the endometrium. There is much controversy about the use of viagra in the UK, and it is not used in all clinics, but its use is common in the US.

The aim at this stage is to try and stay focused on producing lots of good, healthy eggs. Try to stay relaxed and take each day as it comes, not least because getting over-anxious about the results of your scans and tests will release adrenaline into your bloodstream. Make a conscious decision to get rid of negative thoughts as they arise, and use meditation techniques to still an agitated mind.

Women worry that they cannot visualize what their eggs or womb lining might look like, but you can envision these using any images you like. Put pictures in your mind that you understand, that have meaning for you and that you can perceive clearly.

Try, also, to avoid stressful situations, or at least try to find ways to deal with them that cause you the least stress. Spend some time each day sitting quietly and breathing deeply, and remember that rest is vitally important. Put your feet up whenever you can and avoid aerobic exercise and activity, which will direct blood to your extremities when you want a good supply going to your womb and your growing eggs. Even just sitting at your desk or driving a car restricts the flow of *qi* to your abdomen; lying down flat or in a semi-recumbent position for some part of the day is better.

Other tips:

- Get plenty of early nights. Never underestimate the power of sleep and rest to enable your body to adapt, repair and grow.
- Drink plenty of water – 2 to 3 litres a day. Water helps the follicles to grow, whereas alcohol, coffee, tea and stimulants should be avoided.
- Your lower abdomen, the area known in Chinese medicine as the lower *chou*, should be kept warm with *moxa*, hot water bottles or heating pads.
- Have regular acupuncture treatment from an experienced practitioner.
- Use grapefruit, lemon or lime essential oils to uplift your spirits, either in a burner, a warm bath or massage oil.
- Eat warm, nourishing foods.
- Take a daily supplement of DHA.
- Take a good vitamin and mineral supplement containing vitamin E and co-enzyme Q10.
- Use visualization: See what you are trying to achieve here – the

sacral chakra is found at the base of the spine, at the level of the sacrum, and is associated with the water element, which in Traditional Chinese Medicine is associated with the kidneys, which are so important for reproduction. Lie down, close your eyes and feel your muscles relax. Focus on breathing from your abdomen. This is called *dai tian* breathing and is the way we all breathed when we were first born. It helps you to relax and allows the blood and qi to circulate.

- Spend at least 10 minutes a day talking to your partner, telling each other how you are feeling, asking for the support you need. Don't expect your partner to be able to read your mind. Tell him your frustrations and what he can do to help. Don't get resentful, it is negative, and don't expect him to know what to do – he doesn't. Be there for one another.

Egg Collection – The Retrieval Process

Retrieval of the eggs from the follicles is generally done using a vaginal ultrasound probe, which the gynaecologist uses to guide a needle to withdraw an egg from each follicle. The process varies slightly from clinic to clinic, but in all cases you will be sedated.

The length of time retrieval takes will depend on the number of follicles, but it isn't generally a lengthy procedure. Once the egg has been aspirated from the follicle, it is inspected under a microscope and given a grading.

This can be a very anxious time for both you and your partner and you'll be desperate to know 'how many eggs?' You will be told the number straight away – but this is not the crucial consideration. Again, it is quality and not quantity that matters. Don't compare yourself to the woman in the next bed – if she has had 20 eggs retrieved, and you have only nine, don't despair. Not all eggs will fertilize, so at this stage the number of eggs retrieved is no indication of how many embryos might result.

On the evening after retrieval you will start to take progesterone, either by vaginal suppository or injection. This helps to prepare the womb lining for implantation. Not everyone produces sufficient amounts of progesterone on her own. If you go on to get pregnant, you will continue to take progesterone for up to 12 weeks, by which time the placenta will be producing enough on its own. Common side-effects of taking progesterone include nausea, constipation and fluid retention.

Q & As

How will I feel after retrieval?

You will probably feel a little groggy from the sedative, and your ovaries and abdomen may feel swollen and sore. You could experience some abdominal cramping, but this usually passes within 24 hours. There is a slight risk of ovarian hyper-stimulation if a large number of eggs have been removed and the follicles fill up with fluid (see page 328). Contact your doctor immediately if you start to develop symptoms.

Is it normal to spot after retrieval?

You may experience red vaginal spotting for 24 to 48 hours. This is no cause for concern, but if the spotting turns into bleeding (soaking a pad), call your clinic at once.

Tips to Help You Recover after Egg Retrieval

- Rest as much as you can, in preparation for the return of the eggs once they are fertilized. Rest and sleep help the body to recover and heal.
- Take the homoeopathic remedy *arnica 6c* four times a day beginning the day before the procedure, to help prevent soreness and bruising.

- Keep the lower abdomen warm, using a heating pad or hot water bottle.
- Take a supplement of DHA – and remember to keep taking supplements containing vitamin C and vitamin E.
- Take a supplement of co-enzyme Q10, which helps to oxygenate the blood following retrieval.
- Acupuncture can help to prepare the body to receive the embryos.
- As you breathe in, imagine the breath going to your solar plexus. As you breathe out, imagine the stress, worry and discomfort leaving your body. This will help you to relax.

Following egg retrieval, it helps to be able to visualize what's happening, in order to heal the ruptured follicles after egg collection. Very often the more eggs you have had retrieved, the more sore you are likely to be, as the follicles fill with fluid, causing a degree of swelling and tenderness in the ovary. Deep, abdominal breathing helps oxygenate and cleanse the blood, while opening the meridians and allowing your *qi* energy to flow freely.

Spend at least 10 minutes each morning and evening doing positive affirmations, telling yourself that everything is working as it should be. Refuse to dwell on 'What ifs' or negative outcomes. Focus your mind on your womb and visualize it preparing for the transfer of your embryos, your ovaries healing, the swelling reducing, and the womb-lining thickening in preparation for the embryos.

Sperm Collection

In order to fertilize your retrieved eggs, your partner will now have to produce sperm, having abstained from sexual intercourse or masturbation for two to three days. Don't underestimated how nerve-wracking it can be for a man to provide a sample on demand. Having to masturbate into a sterile container, either in the clinic toilet or in a private room furnished with pornography, can be a cold and humiliating experience. If you or your partner have very strong objections to this, it is possible in some cases to get permission to produce a sample at home and then bring it into the clinic. Talk to your doctors about this.

Fertilization

Fertilization protocols vary from clinic to clinic, but a decision will already have been made about the best option for you. This will mean either:

1. IVF (in-vitro fertilization) – the sperm are prepared, washed and counted and then mixed with the eggs in a culture medium in a small shallow dish in the laboratory. If fertilization has taken place, there will be two pronuclei (one nucleus from the egg, one from the sperm). The embryo will be ready for transfer from approximately 48 hours onwards – your clinic will let you know when to come in to have them transferred.

2. ICSI (intra-cytoplasmic sperm injection) – a single sperm is injected into the egg under a microscope, using a fine glass needle.

ICSI is the technique generally used when:

• The sperm parameters are poor and the sperm cannot penetrate the egg on their own.

• The sperm have to be surgically obtained from the testes because there are none present in the ejaculate.

• There has been a poor or non-existent rate of fertilization with previous IVF attempts.

A number of different procedures can be used. If there are enough eggs, IVF and ICSI is carried out in the same treatment cycle by some clinics if they have concerns about fertilization with IVF alone.

AH (assisted hatching) is another procedure, where the outer shell of the egg, known as the zona, is weakened or 'cracked' to help the embryo to 'hatch' and implant. It is commonly used with the eggs of older women, whose shells may have a hardened outer surface.

Once the eggs are retrieved they are put with the sperm for fertilization. Usually you will be contacted and told how many have fertilized. Cell division starts to occur, and your clinic will decide when it is best to transfer the embryos back to your womb. Some clinics will transfer at 2 or 3 days, others will wait for the blastocyst stage (around 5 days after fertilization).

Not all embryos make it to this stage, however, and if not transferred early enough there is a chance that their development might stop, so it is a delicate balancing act to get the timing right. Be guided by your doctor's and embryologist's experience here.

Sometimes you may have good-quality spare embryos stored and frozen from a previous treatment cycle. These can be thawed and transferred to the womb in a natural cycle or with other protocols as decided by your specialist. Not all embryos will survive the thawing process, so there is a reduced success rate, but I have worked with many women who have successfully become pregnant using only one frozen embryo. It is always possible to beat the odds.

Possible Hurdles at This Point

At this stage, there remain some obstacles. Not all eggs will go on to fertilize and divide, for example. This is the main common problem. This may be because they are too immature; they may be too ripe or of poor quality; they may be fertilized by defective sperm or fail to fertilize at all. However, if you have done what you can to support the production of good eggs and sperm, this will help.

Embryo Grading

You will naturally be passionately interested in the quality and development of your embryos, and will probably be asking for regular progress reports. I urge you to remember that the grading of your embryos does not correspond directly to your chances of becoming pregnant. High-grade embryos show a trend towards higher pregnancy rates, but they do not mean pregnancy for certain. I have worked with couples whose grading at every stage was brilliant but who failed to achieve a successful pregnancy, and I have worked with couples who were dependent on one frozen embryo and had a successful birth. So many things come into play, which is why I focus so particularly on a holistic approach, working to promote a good womb lining as well as good eggs and sperm.

Embryo grading helps your doctor determine how many embryos to transfer, but it is a subjective art, not an absolute science. Try to be positive about the embryos that are transferred, regardless of their grading – who knows which one could end up as your baby? Visualize your embryos as having enormous potential and capability, however lowly graded they may be.

To help you visualize what is happening to your embryos, this is the timetable of embryo development (you may also want to take another look at the illustration in the Conception chapter, page 84):

DAY 0: Egg retrieval, sperm collection and preparation, insemination.
DAY 1: The eggs are checked for fertilization and the presence of two pronuclei.
DAY 2: The embryo usually contains between two and four cells. The

first cell division takes place after 36 hours; each successive division then occurs after approximately 12 hours.

DAY 3: The embryo has around 6 to 8 cells.

DAY 4: The embryo contains between 12 and 16 cells and is known as a *morula*.

DAY 5: The embryo has so many cells that individual cells are no longer recognizable; it is now known as a *blastocyst*.

Multi-cell embryos are usually graded from 1 to 4. You may have embryos all of one grade, but are more likely to have embryos from differing grades.

Pre-implantation Genetic Diagnosis

PGD is a technique increasingly being used for testing embryos for genetic disorders before they are transferred into the uterus. Only embryos without abnormalities will be picked for implanting. Around 50 per cent of miscarriages with IVF conceptions occur because of abnormal embryos, so PGD increases your chances of success. It also gives people with serious genetic disorders the chance to minimize the risk of passing on the disorder to their children.

Q & As

How does PGD work?

The most common procedure is for the embryologist, on Day 3 of the embryo's development, to use microscopic instruments to extract one or two cells from each embryo. These cells contain a complete copy of all the embryo's genetic material, and can be analysed for any genetic abnormalities.

Who should consider PGD?

There are a number of reasons to consider PGD:

- those with a racial or ethnic association to specific diseases
- those with specific diseases or genetic disorders running in their families
- those who have had repeated miscarriages.

What can PGD test for?

Currently there are more than 20 diseases that can be tested for, including cystic fibrosis, Huntington's disease, Duchenne Muscular Dystrophy, haemophilia A, Fragile X Syndrome and the propensity to develop breast cancer.

What are the first steps to PGD?

You will be referred to a genetic counsellor and may be given 'carrier testing' to see if there are any specific genetic disease risks already evident. The technology for PGD adds around £2,000 to the cost of IVF. It's also worth remembering that if you are having PGD, it will take five days before the embryos can be transferred.

Transfer of the Embryos

Transfer happens between 48 hours and five days after fertilization, depending on what you and your clinic decide. A number of factors will be considered to decide when the embryos need to be put back. This will depend on the number of available embryos and the quality of the embryos.

It is quite an achievement to have got this far, so be positive and try hard to minimize your inevitable anxiety. Remember that there are no certainties, but it is always possible to beat the odds. I have seen successful pregnancies result from poor quality embryos, frozen embryos and poor sperm.

Your embryos will be loaded into a small flexible catheter, which is inserted through the vagina and cervix into the womb. Some clinics map out your womb in advance, while others use an abdominal ultrasound to guide the embryos into place. When the catheter is in the optimum position near the top of the uterus, the embryos are expelled and the catheter slowly removed. The catheter is then checked back at the lab to make sure there are no embryos remaining inside.

Tips to Prepare for Embryo Transfer

- Lying on your back for a clinical procedure can be stressful, especially when people keep telling you to relax. The adrenaline released by stress could cause your womb to contract, so use whatever relaxation or meditation techniques work for you. Focus on your breathing, welcome the embryos into your body and visualize them floating safely into your nurturing womb.
- If possible, ask to be allowed to watch the procedure on screen, if you feel this will help you to relax and give you a better sense of what is happening to your embryos.
- It can help to have your partner with you, though don't insist if he is reluctant. You need someone with you who can relieve your stress, not add to it.

Q & As

What drugs accompany this stage?

Most clinics will prescribe progesterone (common brand names Crinone or Prometrium) or hCG. These help to sustain a pregnancy, prepare the lining of the womb to accept the fertilized eggs and provide support for the developing embryos.

Progesterone will be given either by intramuscular injection or by vaginal or anal suppository. If implantation is successful, treatment with progesterone may be continued for 10 to 12 weeks, by which time the placenta will be producing enough progesterone itself. Heparin, Ritalin or aspirin are also prescribed by some clinics.

What will the transfer process be like?

This is usually a relatively painless procedure. You will be fully conscious.

How many embryos should I transfer?

Clinics will not allow you to transfer more than two embryos at a time, as the danger of complications rises significantly with a multiple pregnancy. But the quality of your embryos starts to decline as you get older, so transferring more may give you a better chance of success. Find out what the statistics are for your individual clinic, and talk to them – and to your partner – early on, so that you feel comfortable with your decision well before it is time to transfer.

What happens to embryos that are not transferred?

Most clinics can freeze spare embryos (if they are considered good enough) for around five years to use in another round of IVF, avoiding the need to repeat the treatment cycle so far. However, the live birth rate per cycle from frozen embryos is usually lower than for fresh embryo transfers.

Is bed-rest recommended after transfer?

In my opinion, most definitely YES. Putting your feet up, for a minimum of three days, is vitally important. It has not been proven that this will increase your chances of getting pregnant, but I believe you should give those embryos every possible chance to implant. After all you have put yourself through, I think it would be madness to go straight back to work. So do not feel guilty about taking time off and staying in bed.

One of the factors important for successful implantation is good blood flow through the womb lining. Activity diverts blood to your extremities and vital centres, whereas lying down allows for a good flow of blood to the womb. Obviously, for some of my clients where this is not an option, I never make them feel guilty about their decision if they have to go back to work.

When does implantation occur?

The embryo reaches the blastocyst stage five days after fertilization, and starts to break out of its outer shell and begins to implant during the next 48 hours. How soon this happens after transfer depends on the stage of the embryo at transfer.

What factors affect implantation?

Obviously IVF clinics are interested in the reasons why IVF fails. In an unassisted pregnancy, implantation begins 6 or 7 days after fertilization. There are special embryonic cells called 'trophoblasts' that later become the placenta. They begin growing in the uterine lining. When the trophoblast and the uterine lining meet, along with immune cells in the lining, they begin to interact through the mutual exchange of hormone-like substances called 'cytokines'. Depending on the level of some of these cells, they either let the embryo implant or reject it. Various drugs can be used during an IVF cycle to help implantation.

The embryos must be healthy and of good quality, the womb lining (endometrium) must be about 10 mm thick, there must be good blood flow through the endometrium and your body must accept (have no immunological reaction to) the embryos.

What happens next?

There is now a two-week wait before a pregnancy test is taken to determine if implantation has been successful.

The two-week wait

This is the worst two weeks you are likely to spend, constantly worrying whether it has worked or not. In my opinion, women have forgotten how to convalesce, so take this time to nurture yourself, build your strength and recover. Spend time in restful contemplation of the stage to follow, although be prepared for good and bad days over the next fortnight, as you ride yet another emotional roller-coaster full of anxiety, hope and a desperate longing to know the outcome. Providing everything has gone well up to this point, you should allow yourself to be positive and optimistic. Even if this is not your first IVF cycle, you are bound to feel a sense of excitement and anticipation.

During this initial time, avoid the following:
- caffeine, smoking, alcohol, drugs
- heavy lifting
- strenuous exercise and housework (including vacuuming)
- bouncing activities (horse-riding, aerobics)
- sun-bathing, saunas, hot tubs, Jacuzzis
- swimming and hot baths
- sexual intercourse and orgasm.

Post-transfer

After the regular scans and tests of the previous weeks, you may feel lost and alone. Your clinic will offer back-up and you should certainly ring them at any time if you are concerned. A friend (preferably one who has gone through the same experience with a positive outcome) can be a great support, especially if your partner is adopting the pragmatic 'either it's worked or it hasn't' attitude. Many women find that IVF chat rooms are a big help at this point!

You will feel very aware that you are 'carrying' and want to be extremely careful with yourself. Don't feel guilty about taking time off work and taking it easy. Plenty of rest and sleep will give your body the very best chance to repair and adapt to pregnancy. At the very least, lie on the sofa with your feet up as often as you can. Get in a stock of videos, read books you've been meaning to read, sort out old photographs, take up cross-stitch or knitting – anything to distract you!

The Chinese believe that if you focus your mind on a particular area of your body, your *qi* energy will follow. So spend 15 minutes every morning and evening visualizing what is happening inside your womb – the embryos floating safely and preparing to embed in the thick endometrium.

Your body prepares for implantation with a cycle of hormonal stimulation. The ovary continues to produce progesterone, the cells of the blastocyst start to release hCG, the endometrial glands in the womb get bigger and the implantation site becomes swollen with new blood capillaries, all gearing up to nourish that embryo.

- The kidneys, considered in Chinese medicine to play a very important role in reproduction, can quickly become depleted during the IVF process. They are considered especially active between 5 and 7 p.m., so this is a crucial time to rest quietly.
- Deep breathing (see page 186) will help you to relax and enhance the supply of oxygen that reaches your womb.
- Colour can play a significant role in enhancing your mood and balancing your body. Different colours are linked to the chakras or energy centres of the body. Red is associated with fertility, blue can soothe stress and anxiety (it is linked to water and the kidneys in Chinese medicine). Orange is particularly helpful around the time of transfer. Surround yourself with blankets, scarves and flowers in these colours.

- Make sure you eat a diet that is rich in protein, zinc and essential fatty acids, important for cell division, healthy cell membranes and hormone production.
- Take a good multi-vitamin and -mineral supplement and DHA during this time.
- Eat foods rich in selenium, such as brazil nuts, black molasses and herring.

Days 4 to 7 Post-transfer

It is usual to feel very down on at least one of these days. You may be starting to get restless, obsessively thinking about the implantation, desperately looking for signs that everything is going as it should and possibly misinterpreting every symptom as a negative. Sore breasts, mild shooting pains and bloating are all signs that things are going well.

Try to keep yourself as occupied as you can. Go for a leisurely walk or do some gentle yoga. Focusing on the colour blue can be helpful if you feel yourself starting to panic, while breathing and meditation techniques will help you to relax while you visualize those embryos happily settling into their new home.

Try not to bottle things up, but talk your worries through with a friend or your partner, focusing on the positive rather than brooding on the negative. But also try not to get obsessive, and balance the time you spend talking about this with other interests and concerns.

I generally discourage women at this stage from having acupuncture or engaging in any other therapies. Stillness and rest should be your bywords here. Many women find, in any case, that they instinctively retreat into themselves and don't feel like socializing or being out and about too much at this time. Rest, relax, and try to visualize the cells of your embryos healthily dividing in preparation for successful implantation.

Days 7 to 14

The waiting seems to be taking an eternity. Even if you are back at work now, you must still try to take things easy and avoid stressful situations. Only do light work and rest as much as you can. Book a long weekend away, or socialize with friends.

Acupuncture to boost your kidney area can be very beneficial at this stage. Make sure you use an acupuncturist who is experienced in treating women undergoing IVF. Interestingly, one of the relevant points treated on the kidney meridian is called 'the Gate of Life'. If you meditate, take time to do so for at least 20 minutes every day. Do lots of positive visualization. Gentle exercise such as taking a walk, massage, yoga, tai chi or Qi gong is great, but avoid all aerobic exercise for the moment. The blood vessels in your womb need a good oxygen supply for now.

Some women will bleed before Day 10 and get quite shocked by this. It is very common for women with IVF to have some form of bleeding, especially if more than one embryo has been transferred. I know it's so easy to get into a really negative state! During this time there will be occasions when you come crashing down, convinced it hasn't worked. You will be shocked by how hopeless you feel even though you thought you were positive and not getting over-excited about everything. But as I always tell my clients, 'It isn't over until it's over.'

What You May Experience

Every woman's experience is different and there is no standard set of symptoms that will tell you that you are pregnant. However, you may notice the following:

- absolutely no symptoms at all – don't panic!
- bloating and fluid retention
- breast tenderness (one of the side-effects of the progesterone you are taking)

- slight cramping
- pre-menstrual symptoms
- drowsiness and exhaustion
- food aversions
- nausea
- slight bleeding or a brownish discharge. This could be hormonal, the result of an embryo implanting or of an embryo detaching.

It's worth remembering that any of these symptoms could also be the effect of the medications you are taking, or of your body's recovery from the IVF cycle. They could be an indication of an impending period, but equally they could be signs that you are indeed pregnant.

The only way to be sure is to be tested by your clinic. Desperate as you are to know the outcome, it really is better to be advised by your clinic when to do the tests.

The clinic may give you a blood test that also measures levels of hCG (human chorionic gonadotrophin) hormone. Your hCG level will double every 48 hours for the first six weeks of pregnancy, and then every 72 hours for the next two to four weeks. The level peaks at about 8 to 10 weeks and then declines and stays at a lower level for the rest of the pregnancy. Even the most sensitive blood test available cannot detect hCG until around 10 days after ovulation, and there is huge variation in the 'normal' hCG level. Pregnancies which will miscarry or which are ectopic (where the embryo implants outside the uterus) often show normal levels initially, while women with low levels may go on to have a healthy pregnancy. If you have been given an hCG injection as part of your fertility treatment, this will make measuring your levels more tricky, as trace amounts can remain in your system for as long as 10 days after injection. If this is the case, two blood tests can be done on separate days. If the level does increase on the second test, the likely chances are that you pregnant.

If the results from the clinic test are positive, many congratulations. Your longed-for goal has been reached. But be prepared to feel a whole range of conflicting emotions as you contemplate the distance you still have to travel. Many women expect to be elated and cannot understand why they feel low and anxious, but this is completely normal. Take a moment to relax and step back to celebrate quietly before you are hit by the next wave of anxieties and concerns.

If your test is negative, do not despair. Although you may feel at your lowest ebb, the experience you have just gone through has not been wasted. It will tell your clinic a great deal about your body's physiology and what is needed for the next attempt.

If you are keen to keep going and have another try, arrange a meeting with your doctor and talk through what has been learned. I have seen many women who have had a failed cycle but go on to conceive naturally the following month.

When IVF Fails

If you feel that you cannot put yourself through another cycle, talk to your doctor about your other options – and be flexible and prepared to move the goal posts if necessary.

As mentioned, IVF challenges every relationship. For many couples I see for whom IVF hasn't worked, it's a gradual disappointment, a 'slow-motion shock'. Women in particular can be devastated when a treatment hasn't worked. Very often many women are over-optimistic about IVF working the first time, but it's worth remembering that the first time gives the clinic a basis for measuring their response to the drugs, which can be built on for the next cycle.

For some couples the temptation is to want to start again as soon as possible. Some women, in particular, feel that if they throw enough money and energy at the problem, they may stand a better chance of success. It's important at this point to have a meeting with your clinician to decide what to do and how best to get yourself fit and ready to start again, if that's what you want and what's best for you and your partner.

Many of the emotions couples feel are on the surface and very raw, and very often they don't know how to deal with them. They want to blame someone; they feel angry and frustrated. Don't get into 'If I had done this' or 'If you had done that'. It is horrible entering this dark place – you feel alone and devastated, you don't want to talk to anyone, you feel hopeless and helpless and fearful. You will only get out of the dark place when you are sick and tired of being in there.

So, if IVF doesn't work, talk about it for no more than three days. Remember – and I'm generalizing here – men talk about it once and then feel they have dealt with it. They may find it of limited value going over the whole thing, and don't express themselves the way women do.

Remember that coming through the other side with your relationship intact is a success, not a failure. Some of the women I see, sadly, can't come out of the dark place; they cannot let go and would rather lose their relationship than stop having IVF. Other couples stay close despite it all. How do you know if your relationship is suffering? If you think it is, then it is. Keep talking, that is what is important.

Moving On

Sometimes I see couples who have made several attempts and are feeling demoralized. You need to be able to feel with each attempt that something different is being done to better your chances. Are you happy with the clinic? Most couples go back following a failed attempt, to discuss what will happen next time. If a clinic is carrying on with the same regime and protocol time after time, think about changing clinics.

Nowadays many clinics are looking closely at the reasons why IVF fails and using different drug regimes. While some are still considered controversial, I have seen many successes for women who have repeatedly miscarried and have had many failed IVF attempts.

While couples often seem to want support to continue, sometimes it's my feeling that what they really need is 'permission' to stop. When this is the case, I provide a re-assessment of the clinical details, a full understanding of their implications, and often a forum for a couple to come to terms with never getting pregnant. Often one partner reaches this conclusion earlier than the other, but feels unable to 'give up' for fear of letting the other down or hurting their feelings.

Deciding to move on can be very painful, and depends on how far you are prepared to go to have a baby. Some will stop at IVF; others will move on to egg donation, surrogacy and adoption.

For those who decide to move on to egg donation there is generally a long waiting list. The positive news is that there is a 60 to 80 per cent chance of a live birth. Also, you do not have to make a rapid decision; you are not up against the clock. Some of the women I see are not ready straight after several failed IVF cycles, naturally enough. They may come back a year or two later when they feel they are ready to go down the egg-donation route. Obviously you will need counselling and support. Preparation for egg donation – physical, emotional and psychological – is something your clinic will help you to cope with.

pregnancy

Congratulations – you're pregnant! Whether or not this has come as a surprise or it has been hard-won, every woman tends to feel a mix of emotions. Many of my clients expect to feel elated, having waited so long for this to happen. Those who have had IVF may have expected to be over the moon, and are surprised when they are not. Relief for some, ambivalence for another, and anxiety too – all these emotions are normal.

You will be aware of absolutely everything that is going on in your body – every twinge, every ache, however slight. Many women convince themselves that this is the end, running to the toilet every five minutes looking for any sign of bleeding. This can be especially difficult for women who have had IVF, where bleeding does tend to be more common. Don't read books that will terrify you. Just try to be positive – easier said than done, I know.

I try to encourage women to rest as much as possible in the early days. Try to take things easy, come home early from work, put your feet up and get some early nights.

It can't be anything other than an emotional time, so don't underestimate the variety of emotions you may feel.

It is very hard for women today: They have to work, get used to what is happening in their bodies and also have so many questions and anxieties. Also, many don't see their doctors or midwives until they are around 12–16 weeks' pregnant.

You may choose to keep the news to yourself, confiding only in your partner and close family and friends, until after the first 12 weeks when you can be more confident of everything proceeding well. There is always a small risk of miscarriage for any woman during the first three months, and for those women who have miscarried before, it is an anxious time. You never quite relax into a pregnancy until you get beyond the point of where you miscarried before. However, by the time of your first routine ultrasound scan, where you will be reassured by your baby's activity and heartbeat, you will probably feel more confident about sharing your news and making plans for the next year of your life.

Testing Times

You can test for pregnancy, with a shop-bought urine test, as soon as your period is late. These tests are pretty accurate and, although you occasionally get a false-negative (so test again a few days later if your period has still not come), you won't get a false-positive result. Try testing first thing in the morning, when the accumulation of pregnancy hormones in the urine is likely to be higher. The pregnancy test is sensitive to the presence of human chorionic gonadotrophin (hCG) hormone in the urine. This is produced from seven days after fertilization, but it takes another seven days or so to produce enough for it to show up in a urine test. So testing *after* your period was due is usually fine.

If your pregnancy is the result of assisted conception, for example IVF, you may be offered a blood test, which will show the presence of hCG earlier than a urine test, before your period is due. Whether or not you are offered this is down to the policy of the fertility unit where your treatment was carried out. This test is sensitive enough to pick up levels of hCG, which may show that while fertilization has occurred, implantation has been delayed or is not happening. A re-test may be recommended.

Signs and Symptoms

If you have been pregnant before, whatever the outcome, you may well be aware of those signs and symptoms of early pregnancy that are specific to you. For some women, swollen breasts may be the first sign as the hormone progesterone kicks in to support the pregnancy. Another woman may feel sick, while another may just feel overwhelmingly tired.

The range of early symptoms which may give you an indication that you are pregnant are:
- tender breasts that may also be swollen
- an increased need to urinate
- feeling nauseous
- vomiting
- increased sensitivity to food tastes, and smells
- enormous feeling of tiredness
- heightened emotions.

However, although these feelings may indicate pregnancy, the only sure way is to do a pregnancy test.

Seeing Your GP

Once you know you are pregnant, you will need to see your GP to discuss what the options are for you for antenatal care in your area. Most areas operate a system of 'shared care' between the GP practice, community midwives and hospital consultant, with the understanding that you will opt to give birth in the consultant or midwife unit of your local hospital. This is likely to be the case if you are considered a 'high-risk' pregnancy. A high-risk pregnancy is determined partly by your age and past gynaecological or obstetric history. However, at this early stage, your best bet is to get booked in and review your options if necessary as you proceed.

Antenatal Tests

While the assumption is made that a pregnancy is normal until shown to be otherwise, a number of antenatal tests are routinely offered, from blood tests for anaemia to ultrasound and to amniocentesis if you are over a certain age. Some tests are designed to monitor your health, and by extension the health of your baby, while other tests are designed specifically to assess the risk of various congenital abnormalities, like Down's Syndrome, in your baby. Discuss the tests with your midwife or doctor so you are aware of what the implications are. For example, if a routine blood test identifies a high risk of Down's Syndrome, you may be offered amniocentesis, which has a risk of miscarriage and may result in the offer of a late termination. This is a worst-case scenario, but it's worth being aware of what the outcome of certain tests might be for a longed-for baby.

What You Can Do

Although it isn't very fashionable to say so, I recommend that women rest as much as they can during the first few months of pregnancy. I also recommend that they drink no alcohol – although I believe a little of what you fancy when you are trying is OK, I believe that in pregnancy all alcohol is feto-toxic.

Women often panic in the early days of pregnancy that they are not eating well, as they have gone off the healthy diet they were eating when they conceived. Many women crave carbs and cannot understand it because they think that they are going to put pounds and pounds of weight on. Don't panic. You need carbs for energy and your body will start to crave them. It takes time in the early days of pregnancy to know how much energy your body needs and how to control it. Try to eat regularly; this will help. I get all of my women on Vital Essence One: it contains 1 gram of vitamin C and 400 iu of vitamin E to help to prevent miscarriage, also vital DHA – eight out of ten woman are deficient in this prior to getting pregnant and you need it for brain and spine development.

You probably will have been taking a pre-conception supplement containing folic acid; continue to do so. Avoid caffeine, alcohol, tobacco, strenuous exercise and hot baths, saunas or steam rooms. I also suggest that sexual intercourse is avoided during the first 12 weeks, although there is nothing to stop couples being sexually intimate in other ways. Nor do I encourage flying in the first trimester, especially long-haul flights. A short course of acupuncture can help ensure that kidney energy is strong, and help relieve any early pregnancy symptoms like nausea and tiredness.

My Programme

My programme starts the minute a woman has a positive pregnancy test result with an early pregnancy health check. It seems that there are so many fears around childbirth these days; it really makes me feel sad, as I believe and have seen a lot of proof of the fact that if a woman feels supported she can get through anything.

Fertility chart

Name _____

Age _____

Chart No. _____

Length of shortest cycle = day ☐   minus 20 = ☐ is first fertile day   Length of this cycle = ☐ days

Route of temperature ☐ O ☐ V ☐ R   Time of taking temperature ☐

Comments

Month & Year			
Date			
Day			

°C: 37.4, 37.3, 37.2, 37.1, **37.0**, 36.9, 36.8, 36.7, 36.6, 36.5, 36.4, 36.3, 36.2, 36.1, **36.0**, 35.9, 35.8, 35.7, 35.6, 35.5

Day of cycle: 1 2 3 4 5 6 7 8 9 10 11 12 13 14 15 16 17 18 19 20 21 22 23 24 25 26 27 28 29 30 31 32 33 34 35 36 37 38 39 40

Sexual Intercourse – Circle day of cycle

Cervical secretions – Wet, slippery, transparent, stretchy

(Feel/look & touch)   Moist, white, cloudy, sticky

Dry, no secretions seen or felt

Period

Cervix
- High, soft, open
- Low, firm, closed
- Tilted or straight

Technology
- Result
- Test day

useful contacts

Fertility

Zita West Clinic
43 Devonshire Street
London W1G 7AL

Zita West Products
Zita West offers a range of
supplements for pre-conception,
fertility and IVF treatment, including
Vitafem, Vitamen and the vital DHA.
www.zitawest.com

**Fertility UK – the National
Fertility Awareness & Natural
Family Planning Service**
www.fertilityuk.org

British Fertility Society
www.britishfertilitysociety.org.uk

**HFEA – the Human Fertilisation
& Embryology Authority**
www.hfea.gov.uk

RELATE – relationship advice
www.relate.org.uk

**British Infertility Counselling
Association**
www.bica.net

Infertility Network
www.infertilitynetworkuk.com

National Infertility Support Network
www.child.org.uk

European Infertility Network
www.ein.org

Donor Conception Network
www.dcnetwork.org

National Gamete Donation Trust
www.ngdt.co.uk

**NIAC – National Infertility
Awareness Campaign**
www.repromed.co.uk/niac/info

Surrogacy UK
www.surrogacyuk.org

IVF
www.ivf.net
www.IVFconnections.com (US)

**ACeBabes – for families
following assisted conception**
www.acebabes.co.uk

Multiple Births Foundation
www.multiplebirths.org.uk

**TAMBA – Twins & Multiple
Births Association**
www.tamba.org.uk

Health and Nutrition

Food Standards Agency
www.foodstandards.gov.uk

British Nutrition Foundation
www.nutrition.org.uk

**Royal College of Obstetricians
and Gynaecologists**
www.rcog.org.uk

Well-being
www.wellbeing.org

Mothers Over 35
www.mothers35plus.co.uk

Women's Health
www.womens-health.co.uk

Miscarriage Association
www.miscarriageassociation.org.uk

National Endometriosis Society
www.endo.org.uk

**Verity – the Polycystic Ovary
Syndrome self-help group**
www.verity-pcos.org.uk

**Daisy Network – for women
with premature menopause**
www.daisynetwork.org.uk

Complementary Therapies

British Complementary Medicine Association
www.bcma.co.uk

British Acupuncture Council
www.acupuncture.org.uk

British Medical Acupuncture Society
www.medical-acupuncture.co.uk

National Institute of Medical Herbalists
www.nimh.org.uk

Society of Homeopaths
www.homeopathy.co.uk

Manual Lymphatic Drainage
www.mlduk.org.uk

British Osteopathic Association
www.osteopathy.org

International Institute of Reflexology
www.reflexology-uk.co.uk

Shiatsu Society
www.shiatsu.org

index